D0491268

How to Lead a Happier, Healthier, Alcohol-Free Life

The Rise of the Soberista

Lucy Rocca

This book is dedicated to all the Soberistas in the world

Published by Accent Press Ltd 2014

ISBN 9781783756117

Foreword by Della Galton

Drinking too much is a problem of our time. And being a woman who drinks too much is still a taboo in modern society. If a man has one too many and staggers off home to sleep it off he may be the recipient of a few sympathetic titters. But if a woman slides off her bar stool and passes out on the floor we are much less forgiving. It's hard to be a woman who drinks too much.

I know because I was one for longer than I care to remember. Making a decision to live life without alcohol was for me, as it is for many women, very difficult. But once I realised I could no longer safely drink, I did make that decision. These last eight years when I have embraced sobriety and all that it means have been the happiest of my life.

If you are starting your alcohol-free journey, one of the most helpful things is to realise that you are not alone. There is a massive amount of support out there. And sharing your experience of going alcohol-free and hearing other people's stories is a very good start.

Lucy Rocca drank too much for most of her adult life. When she gave up she founded the wonderful Soberistas – an online forum where other people who wanted to try life alcohol-free could chat, share their stories, and give each other unconditional support.

How to Lead a Happier, Healthier, Alcohol-Free Life *is her fourth book about quitting drinking. Between the pages of this frank account Lucy explains how she became alcohol-free entirely and found happiness, and how you can do the same thing.*

Here's to you and your alcohol-free life.

With very best wishes

Della Galton
Author of the novel Ice and a Slice
www.dellagalton.co.uk

Sober Syllabification: (so·ber) Pronunciation: /ˈsōbər/

Adjective (soberer, soberest) not affected by alcohol; not drunk.

Serious, sensible, and solemn: a sober view of life his expression became sober
    Free from alcoholism; not habitually drinking alcohol: I've been clean and sober for five years
    Muted in colour: a sober grey suit

Verb

Make or become sober after drinking alcohol: [with object]: that coffee sobered him up [no object]: I ought to sober up a bit
    Make or become more serious, sensible, and solemn: [no object]: his expression sobered her (as adjective sobering) a sobering thought

4

Prologue

"Hit the bottom and get back up; or hit the bottle and stay down."
   – Anthony Liccione

I defined myself by my dependency on alcohol for twenty years. I was a wino, a boozer, a good-time girl. Nights out did not happen unless they were structured around drinking; nights in spent not under the influence were hours wasted, time to get out of the way before the real living began once more and another bottle was opened.

Holidays presented an extended opportunity to drink minus the constraints of the normal working week. Weekends when my daughter stayed with her dad constituted forty-eight hours of alcoholic indulgence, beginning in the pub on Friday after work and concluding at 5 p.m. Sunday, the last glass being drained just seconds before she arrived home.

There were, however, a few obstacles standing in the way of my bottles of chilled pinot grigio and true happiness. When I had my last alcoholic drink I was thirty-five and my daughter Isobel was twelve years old. For the duration of her childhood, her mum had 'liked a drink'. Much of this boozing had occurred when she was either in bed or at her dad's house, but the consequences of too much alcohol lay all around for her to witness; my mood swings, lethargy and hangovers, ditching the car after Sunday lunch in a pub and calling a taxi instead because Mummy had had too much to safely get behind the wheel, strangers asleep on the settee, invited to spend the night

5

after several bottles had been drunk into the early hours of the morning as Isobel slept peacefully and blissfully unaware upstairs.

And here lay the first (and biggest) reason for my questioning a growing dependence upon wine – I felt guilty, and was all too conscious of the fact that my alcohol misuse would (if it hadn't already done so) have a damaging impact on Isobel's state of mind, negatively affecting her sense of security and our future mum/daughter relationship. In addition to the concerns that I felt with regards to Isobel's wellbeing (and how my alcohol consumption threatened that) during my latter drinking years I also developed an increased awareness of the state of my own health and how booze was putting my body at risk of God knows how many scary conditions.

Breast cancer, cirrhosis, death by drunkenness, early onset dementia – I wasn't stupid and I knew full well that the writing was on the wall for any number of the above health consequences (and plenty more), should I choose to maintain my longstanding wine habit.

The result of these fears over my excessive boozing was that I eventually made the decision to quit alcohol altogether, for ever. Perennially unable to moderate, I realised that, if I continued as I was, my entire time on the planet would come to be defined by my drunkenness. My daughter's emotional security, my reputation, my appearance, my achievements (or lack of), my relationships, my self-esteem, and how I viewed the world; it would all amount to nothing more than the sum total of too many nights spent drunk. I wanted, and needed, much more than that – for both of us.

Now, here's the dilemma I found myself faced with: the opposite of being drunk is sobriety. My biggest issue in making this choice to adopt a pure existence was that I couldn't imagine myself as a person who shuns letting her hair down in favour of quiet nights drinking mineral water, perpetually looking after herself, regularly sleeping eight hours, and parting company from the crowd of party animals that had generated my entire adult social life. I was carving out a future based on clean living; never again would I be the reckless, wayward rebel.

What would I be? Who would I become? The years ahead stretched out like an endless road of monotony. No crises, car-crash situations, or doomed relationships based on boozing; no more mornings spent hiding in bed, crippled by debilitating hangovers, or impetuous weekends away booked at 1 a.m. with wine glass in one hand and plastic fantastic in the other. I would never again experience false, alcohol-induced confidence or shameful hours spent lying on the settee with mascara streaked across cheeks and fear in the pit of the stomach. All of this would be consigned to the memory bin and day-to-day life suddenly offered nothing more than good sense and self-confidence. Over the years I had grown dependent, not only on alcohol, but on a warped and negative way of being. My adult history was littered with bad choices and low emotions, and I had never known true self-esteem since childhood. I felt unanchored at the mere thought of life without my gloom and mayhem.

My musical heroes were Anthony Kiedis of the Red Hot Chili Peppers and Shaun Ryder of the Happy Mondays. I listened to the Stone Roses, Nirvana, any good dance music of the late 1980s/1990s, Joy Division, New Order, Johnny Cash, and Oasis – bands that lent themselves to indulging in the rock and roll lifestyle, artists who sang about drugs and addiction and the dark side. I understood their lyrics and outlook. I felt a part of what these people stood for. *I* was rock n roll, for God's sake.

My biggest worry rested on the notion that without alcohol I would be dull, that as a non-drinker I could no longer realistically present myself as a free-thinker, a rebel, a person who rejects conformist attitudes. I desperately wanted to retain the version of me that consumed alcohol in excessive quantities, smoked Marlboro Lights, and clung to these addictive substances in the visceral belief that, somehow, they made me worthy. I have to be honest; for a long time, I hated the thought of never drinking again.

And yet, sobriety it had to be.

At no stage did I feel content with the idea of living as the kind of teetotaller who grits her teeth to make it through each alcohol-craving day, longing for a cold glass of pinot grigio but forced to put up with a Diet Coke instead. No, that would never do. I wanted to think like a person who had *never* been troubled by alcohol issues, the type who might indulge in the odd sherry at Christmas but who is then perfectly happy with nothing alcoholic to drink for the rest of the year. I needed to fall *out* of love with booze and in love with, well, *me*.

Sober living means no façades behind which to hide. It means knowing who you are inside and out, liking that person, and never feeling the urge to run screaming into the arms of your (drunken) alter ego. Being straight all of the time removes the cheat's route to feeling relaxed, it presents many spare hours all of a sudden, and asks that they be filled with *stuff*. Sobriety forces the issue of sex minus the (for many) convenient fog of inebriation – getting naked sober takes balls! Living alcohol-free smashes through ALL the bullshit and demands a person face life head-on.

I wasn't sure that any of that appealed, back in April 2011. Alcohol had definitely helped induce sexual confidence in me. It was my most reliable prop when it came to socialising amongst people I was not overly familiar with, and it happily brought about a metamorphosis from boring to fun, no matter which teeth-pulling situation I may have found myself in.

Drinking, not to put too fine a point on it, made me into the person I was. I was a Drinker. Take away the ethanol and I feared for a while that I might just wither away and disappear into thin air. And thrown into the jumble of all this anxiety was the creeping suspicion that maybe, just maybe, life was pretty pointless.

Far harder than coming to terms physically with the notion of never having a drink again, was accepting the idea of becoming a person who does not drink. Ever since my early teens I had defined myself as a rebel, a defiant individual who permanently held two fingers up to authority. Getting drunk, in my mind, slotted right in with this self-image and I could not conceive of a life devoid of the prop that I imagined formed the central core of my personality. People who behaved themselves and accepted a quiet life staying in to watch the soaps with a cup of tea, maintaining a pristine home that shines as brightly as their reputation, and always obtaining a solid eight hours of sleep were the ones who I associated with the alcohol-free lifestyle. Car-washing at 8 a.m. on a Sunday, striving for promotions at work, looking out for their neighbours, and showing their face in church on a regular basis – this was the crowd that I envisaged I was joining, but I couldn't imagine my living their existence one little bit.

When non-sympathisers accuse heavy drinkers of irresponsibility and call for them to control their urges and sort themselves out, they fail to recognise that for many it is precisely the irresponsible and reckless nature of excessive alcohol consumption that draws certain people towards it in the first place. We like the fact that we don't conform; we enjoy the fighting spirit that we feel is conveyed by our indulgent drinking habits. The last thing we want to do is quit drinking and act responsibly, as this would be tantamount to losing all sense of the person we are.

The society we live in can make it incredibly difficult

and unappealing to contemplate an alcohol-free life for three major reasons: a) alcohol is generally revered all over the Western hemisphere, b) the alcohol industry is given something of a free rein when it comes to marketing and advertising its products, and c) those who are teetotal are largely regarded as boring; people frequently associate sobriety with overly religious types who have a desire to convert the masses into grey and joyless do-gooders.

But what happens when you are just a normal person who has always loved getting pissed and you are suddenly floored (for whatever reason) with the realisation that you cannot drink any more (that is, if you wish to cling on to your dignity, family, and liver)? How does one go about navigating ones way through the sparkling and full-of-health world of sober living? How do you get, and stay, sober?

In order for me to deal with my earth-shattering decision to quit drinking (and to commit to such a radically new way of living) it was essential that I get my head around sobriety. I wanted to fully understand exactly why I had come to rely on booze so heavily, and what it was about alcohol-free life that I was so dismissive and afraid of. I needed to fit as comfortably with *non*-drinking as I had with knocking back a bottle a night (on a quiet evening); I needed to like the idea of me, sober.

This book, then, provides an in-depth look at sobriety. It examines why, as a society, we take such issue with it while simultaneously holding alcohol in such high regard. It looks at self-image and how, as we grow up, alcohol frequently becomes such a key factor in the way we perceive ourselves and how we live. The book highlights historical figures associated with sobriety, and examines the alcohol-free life in a practical and realistic way, focusing on what it really means to not drink in the contexts of sex, body confidence, socialising, and friendships.

How to Lead a Happier, Healthier, Alcohol-Free Life details the trajectory of women throughout the latter half of the twentieth century and into the new millennium, and how the birth of the 'ladette' culture together with powerful marketing and advertising strategies by the wine industry have resulted in many Western women of all ages increasing their alcohol consumption in the belief that they are indulging in a treat. It investigates the idea that alcohol-free living *can* equate to being cool, and why quitting drinking does not have to mean transforming one's character from fun-lover to dullard.

As a person who spent more than twenty years almost surgically attached to a bottle of wine, it was vital for my sanity that I learnt to love being sober with a passion equal to that which I'd felt towards booze. And to fall in love with anything, one has to familiarise oneself with it first – this then, is your comprehensive guide to the world of sobriety.

Chapter One – Maslow's Wisdom

"We are what we pretend to be, so we must be careful about what we pretend to be."
  – Kurt Vonnegut

At some stage between the age of twelve and thirteen and a half, I developed a crush on alcohol. As the transformation began to occur from conscientious schoolgirl to wayward and rebellious teenager, I silently and unwittingly acknowledged the fact that I was going to become a drinker.

December 1988, a Christmas party; my family and I arrived at the hosts' house (friends of my parents) and mingled politely amongst the already-present guests. It didn't take long before my friend and I discovered the extended table in the dining room which was simply groaning with bottles of booze. As Kylie Minogue played loudly from the hi-fi in the corner, we embarked (in expert fashion, despite it being the first time either of us had sipped anything more potent than a thimbleful of white wine with Sunday lunch) on the act of getting pissed.

The Martinis were poured, cocktail umbrellas added to make everything yet more fancy and grown-up, and off we danced into a state of inebriation. Meanwhile, oblivious to our shenanigans, my parents were chattering away to their friends and sipping alcoholic beverages in a responsible style elsewhere in the house. Eventually, when our drunken states were reported to them we were dragged off the premises and marched home with our tails between our legs.

What I remember most vividly though about the whole episode took place the following morning in the kitchen when my grandma, with whom we lived, shook her head in disdain as I staggered past her clutching my head (in order to illustrate the fact that I had a hangover). I chuckled and said breezily, "Oh come on Granny – what's Christmas about if not to get pissed!" Unsurprisingly my grandma gasped and looked at me with an expression that said: "You cheeky, precocious little shit" and proceeded to viciously attack a pile of potatoes with her peeling knife.

What does this incident reveal about me, a typical middle-class teenager of the late eighties, and the unbelievably normalised face of excessive alcohol consumption? I was not, during my childhood, exposed to extreme alcohol misuse, addiction to other drugs, or violence or abuse of any sort. A few months previously I had spent most of my spare time either playing with Sindy dolls, reading Enid Blyton books, or writing short stories. And yet, somehow, this innocent youth gave way very rapidly to a desire to obliterate my world as often as possible through the use of alcohol.

I often wonder whether I was born to be wild and thus all the drinking and partying was merely the manifestation of me finding my feet on the predestined path of Lucy's life. Or alternatively, was I actually fairly sensible, whereby the excessive boozing and other debauched antics were evidence of how I was blown, quite catastrophically, off course by alcohol?

My character as a child was somewhat bolshie. A leader and organiser (whether my friends enjoyed these aspects of my personality is another matter – I have been labelled 'bossy' more times than I care to remember in my life!) I was not one to hide away in the corner. Throughout my school life I had many friends and, later on, boyfriends. I was hard-working and creative, and I exuded confidence and self-assurance. Beneath the surface, however, I remember experiencing frequent moments of self-doubt; I would have 'wobbles' and worry that I didn't fit in.

I recall one lunchtime at primary school being taught how to make a pot of tea by a teacher. A friend and I had been selected to watch over the biscuits our class had made in the previous lesson and which were baking in the ovens, and the teacher suggested showing us how to make a pot of tea as a way of passing the time. Aged about seven, I'd never been near a kettle before and had absolutely no clue as to how one goes about making tea. I watched intently and listened conscientiously, gearing up for the chance to have a go myself. The teacher left the classroom for a few minutes leaving us to it, and that's where it all got quite confused in my head. I added the leaf-tea, not to the teapot but inside the kettle, which I then filled with water and switched on to boil.

When the teacher returned and witnessed my bungled attempt at tea-making, she burst into peals of laughter which continued for what seemed like hours. I laughed it off brazenly but inside I was utterly crushed and desperately wanted to run screaming from the school and never return. I was (and still am) an utter perfectionist and couldn't bear the thought that I'd slipped up and made such a clumsy error while undertaking an apparently simple task.

That feeling of inferiority returned over and over again throughout my childhood, teens, and twenties. One time, as a Brownie Guide, I was instructed to make a decorative item from fabric during the forthcoming week, in order to obtain my 'Craft Badge'. My fellow Brownies all returned the following session bearing extravagant and sophisticated creations which wouldn't have looked out of place in John Lewis's soft furnishings department. It was obvious that their parents had helped out considerably with this particular task. My heart sank as I gazed around at my friends' offerings, comparing them unfavourably with my own 1-D ragged piece of felt, cut roughly into a house shape (it was weak, I'll be honest, but at least it was my own work!)

The Brown Owl (leader of the Brownie group) proceeded to dangle my 'house' in front of the other girls who all fell about in fits of hysterics, and that familiar sensation of churning stomach and self-loathing flooded my whole being once again.

Meanwhile, as these and other incidents occurred periodically during my youth, I continued to project a confident, almost cocksure, attitude, and those around me more than likely had no idea of the extent to which I beat myself up inside. Low self-esteem is often disguised through the presentation of different 'faces' to the outside world. There are the people who act full of bravado, loudly vocalising their achievements to anyone who will listen, but who are riddled with the secret fear that they'll be found out for who they really are; an imposter. There are the rebellious ones who portray an attitude of not caring, the type of person who demonstrates aggression and anger as their default position. And there are the victims, people severely lacking in self-confidence and the ability to make their own decisions, who rely on self-pity in the hope that others will help them out, never making an effort to work through things independently.

It was a mixture of these three personas which formed the disguise of my own increasingly low self-esteem as I matured through my teenage years. Cocky, arrogant, and loud, but occasionally consumed by utter helplessness and self-pity, I unwittingly allowed those early fleeting moments of self-doubt to creep up on me and become a real part of who I was.

Looking back, I believe that the fact I did not acknowledge (even to myself) those feelings of inadequacy contributed greatly to my desire to get drunk. Alcohol not only makes us forget, it also buoys us up with Dutch courage, providing a false but seemingly very real sense of confidence. For someone who is being gently eaten away inside by her insecurities but who cannot admit this to anyone, alcohol appears to be the perfect medicine.

Teenagers are at a particularly high risk of falling for the myth that alcohol is a magical substance which injects confidence and glamour like nothing else, as they have very little, if any, grasp of their own mortality. For a person who imagines they will live for ever, the warnings related to excessive alcohol consumption mean absolutely nothing. James Dean once said 'Dream as if you'll live for ever. Live as if you'll die today', and for most teenagers, me included, this is exactly the way to go.

So what is self-esteem and why is it so tightly woven with the issue of alcohol consumption? A healthy self-esteem means having the strength of character to bat off life's difficulties without crumbling under their weight. It results in the ability to avoid perceiving every problem as if it were a personal affront. When one is lacking in self-esteem, feelings of inadequacy and inferiority rise to the surface and prevent a person from fulfilling their true potential.

I speak from many years of personal experience when I say that a couple of alcoholic drinks work well, and fairly dramatically, at diluting these negative emotions – in the immediate and very short term at least. The problems come about over a period of time, and are insidious in the way they are realised.

Aged twenty, I fell in love with a drug dealer. He was a 'recovered' heroin addict although he had merely swapped one drug (heroin) for another (legal) one: alcohol. My relationship with this man was the perfect illustration of how a person with low self-esteem becomes trapped in a cycle of negativity, a self-fulfilling prophecy which is all-too-often spurred along by booze. He was a drinker, I was a drinker. We met in a pub frequented by heavy drinkers; it's fair to say that during that period of my life, I was awash with booze.

Our social life revolved around the pub in which we met and from the very beginning we fell into a pattern of meeting, drinking, arguing, passing out, and doing it all over again the next day when we woke up. I thought I was Nancy to his Sid Vicious. I was in love with the excitement of being so bad, and I believed I was in love with him. On reflection I view his effect on me as being similar to that of alcohol; in short bursts of fun and recklessness he made me feel overwhelmed with love and happiness, but over any significant length of time my mood would be low far more often than it was high. I was frightened of my reaction to him, and yet I kept returning for another dose of the same.

He put me down in very subtle ways and incrementally chipped away at my friendships until I spent almost all my time with him, drunk. I did everything he said, and defended him to the bitter end. The relationship was doomed to end badly, and after several months it did exactly that. Quite suddenly I came to my senses and finished with him, feeling as though I needed to escape before I found that I couldn't. He did not take kindly to me ending things, and his reluctance to let go culminated in me having him arrested in the early hours of one summer's morning for assault and battery, breaking and entering, and false imprisonment.

Thankfully I regained a grip on normality and we drifted apart, our paths never crossing again. However, I often think of that man as personifying the terribly innocuous-seeming hold that alcohol can have over us, and as illustrating how we can easily fall madly in love with something so dangerous and detrimental to our wellbeing.

The Scottish philosopher, Thomas Carlyle (1795–1881)

once said, "Nothing builds self-esteem and self-confidence like accomplishment" and I firmly believe that this is one of the key reasons why alcohol retains its vice-like control over us, even when we know it is causing us so much harm. The simple fact is that when we are drinking heavily and regularly, we don't accomplish anything of much substance, in fact, the opposite is true; drinking away our evenings results in us undoing elements of our lives in which we have *already* accomplished something, be it our relationships with partners, children, or friends, our careers, financial security, health and fitness, or our reputations.

Successful relationships, regardless of who they are with, demand effort, self-sacrifice, and a good degree of self-awareness. Long-term, excessive alcohol consumption plays havoc with all of these qualities, resulting in an inability to fully possess any one of them. Without self-esteem it is virtually impossible to be truly self-aware, and self-sacrifice is a difficult concept to grasp when one is caught up in feelings of inferiority and a victim complex.

In all the relationships I was involved in as a drinker I was unable to accept criticism, flying off the handle for the most trivial of matters. I would internalise my irritations and anger, powerless to vocalise my emotions in a constructive way, and after every major row I would merely drink the problem away. Although I hate to point the finger solely at alcohol (I did, after all, lift each glass and drink from it), I feel quite certain that a) I probably wouldn't have ended up with any of my past partners had booze not played its part, and b) if, in the unlikely scenario that I had wound up dating any of my exes as a non-drinker, the arguments, jealousies, misunderstandings, and infidelities would never have occurred. Almost all the negative aspects of my past relationships came about because I had zero self-esteem, which in turn was largely as a consequence of the amount of alcohol I was consuming.

Being in possession of adequate self-esteem allows us to understand whether we are being treated with respect. It provides us with the mental tools we require to recognise when we are in the right, and when we have acted out of turn. Crucially, the possession of self-esteem means that we don't take criticism to heart and react badly to it, but are able to utilise it in a helpful way to learn from our mistakes and better ourselves.

Having self-awareness equates to knowing who we are, inside and out. We are able to acknowledge where our weaknesses lie and what our strengths are; we have a deep understanding of ourselves which enables us to make conscious change in our lives, where change needs to be made. Self-awareness helps motivate us to alter negative habits and provides us with the drive to switch course and do things differently and better. Breaking out of bad habits is only possible when we are able to recognise the detrimental effects a habit is having in our lives – being self-aware affords us the understanding that a particular future we may crave cannot be ours unless we stop acting in a certain way.

Self-awareness, put simply, is the passport to self-fulfilment, and it is virtually impossible to possess when we are caught up in a destructive cycle of heavy alcohol consumption. Being aware of our every facet can only occur when our self-esteem is buoyant – without self-esteem we perceive ourselves and those around us with a warped vision.

My life as a drinker was very small in comparison to the way it is today. The horizons of my existence were no broader than my next alcoholic drink, although when I was caught up in the booze trap I had no comprehension of this being the case – I firmly believed that all my desires were my own and did not stem from the need to obtain my next fix of alcohol. Prior to being a parent my evenings were almost always spent in the pub, and should I have stayed at home then it would never have been without a decent supply of wine or beer to see me through the evening. Spending each night under the influence resulted in my goals being nothing more substantial than cooking a nice meal (excellent justification for a good bottle of wine, or three) or watching a film.

While these are pleasant enough activities they do not act as self-esteem boosters. We simply do not derive the same kind of satisfaction and pride from catching up, glass to hand, on the latest blockbuster, or rustling up a meal which we then wash down with sense-numbing alcohol, as we do from setting goals which demand real effort and the conquering of obstacles.

Goals that take true effort and self-sacrifice tend to be longer-term in nature than, for instance, viewing a film, but when we drink excessively (and by excessive I mean two or three decent-sized glasses of wine per evening) it's impossible to focus on anything which demands a good degree of brain power. Establishing a business, for example, means weeks if not months of planning; the financial aspects, a solid business plan, staff, marketing, the product itself – it all requires masses of work and organisation, but when the outcome is a successful and flourishing enterprise the rewards are huge, not least to our self-esteem.

Learning a new skill, be it mastering a foreign language, developing an artistic streak or training for a physical challenge like a marathon, takes time, patience, and commitment. When we do not drink and are therefore able to apply ourselves fully to goals we set, we reap the rewards of satisfaction, pride, and fulfilment which all substantially boost self-esteem. However, when we booze away the evenings and our hopes and dreams fall by the wayside, the opposite occurs; our self-esteem plummets and we chastise ourselves, believing we are no good at anything and are in some way inferior to others who seem to achieve so much.

Before I quit drinking I would scoff at those who engaged in hobbies, perceiving them as boring and nerdy. Now I understand that hobbies are so much more than just a way of passing the time, a means of distracting ourselves from the humdrum of life. Hobbies act as an effective method of establishing goals, allowing us to become accomplished at something not everyone can do – yes, hobbies are actually a tool for building self-esteem.

Another means to building self-esteem is through socialising and engaging with people who boost our confidence. Other people can make us feel good about ourselves – being in their company acts as a mirror to our personalities and their reaction to us helps create our self-image. When we are in control of our actions and speech, this can be a good thing – telling a joke, for instance, and seeing our friends fall about laughing is reassuring and an effective sign telling us we are funny and well liked. Being drunk, staggering about, and boring people with the same old story we've told a thousand times but cannot remember due to the effects of alcohol, has the opposite effect.

My self-image deteriorated during the last few years I spent drinking. I was well aware of my reputation as something of a nightmare on nights out. I was the liability who would always have one too many, the one who some well-meaning friend or other would attempt to sober up with a cup of strong coffee while simultaneously steering me away from the bar. I made bad choices, argued with people, reacted in a hostile and over-the-top way to situations that did not necessitate such a response, and flirted outrageously with men to whom I did not actually feel attracted.

The outcome of such behaviours was that my self-image was very poor. In conjunction with this, I gave my self-esteem absolutely no chance to blossom because I rarely set myself goals, and subsequently I achieved very little that I could be proud of. Without any self-esteem, I had absolutely no chance of developing my self-awareness, the one thing that was vital in helping motivate me to change all my bad habits.

Abraham Maslow, the American psychologist most famous for creating his 'Hierarchy of Needs' theory of psychological health, said the following:

"It is quite true that man lives by bread alone – when there is no bread. But what happens to man's desires when there is plenty of bread and when his belly is chronically filled?

"At once other (and 'higher') needs emerge and these, rather than physiological hungers, dominate the organism. And when these in turn are satisfied, again new (and still 'higher') needs emerge and so on. This is what we mean by saying that the basic human needs are organized into a hierarchy of relative prepotency." (Maslow, 1943, p. 375, A Theory of Human Motivation)

Over the decades Maslow amended his hierarchy model but the original version purported that human beings cannot advance to a higher level of need until the following, more basic ones are taken care of; physiological needs (i.e. food, water, warmth) must be addressed prior to a person being able to meet the safety needs of security and freedom from fear. With these in place, we are then able to focus on achieving a sense of belonging (i.e. friends, family, and spouse), and subsequently on attaining self-esteem (achievement, mastery, recognition, and respect). Finally, with all the lower needs taken care of, human beings are capable of self-actualization (are able to pursue inner talent, creativity, and fulfilment).

According to Maslow's model then, once the more basic survival needs have been met, a person should be in a position to focus on the next stage, a sense of belonging.

In reality my belly was mostly full of chablis or pinot grigio, but the scenario is the same; I had my food, water, warmth (and wine), physical security, and safety needs met, and therefore I was able to indulge in some of the more enjoyable, less survival-based, aspects of life – or was I?

Maslow highlighted one of the most basic needs as 'freedom from fear', which he positioned on the same level as security. He maintained that before one could truly be free to move on to the subsequent need of a sense of belonging, one must be without the constraints of worry and anxiety over one's safety. If you are a regular and heavy boozer (and anything like I was as a drinker), then fear will raise its ugly head on a pretty frequent basis in your day-to-day life; fear of never being able to escape the alcohol trap, fear of dying prematurely, fear of how drinking too much might be impacting on your loved ones, fear over what happened last night (which you can't remember due to experiencing yet another blackout), and fear of wasting life.

With all these anxious and negative thoughts whirling around, it is virtually impossible to focus on enjoying a healthy relationship with a partner, or nurturing long-lasting and meaningful friendships. With no self-esteem, a person is likely to feel paranoid, jealous, and be lacking in confidence – traits which are not conducive to establishing and maintaining a happy union with anyone. The chances are that if you are a heavy drinker your partner will enjoy hitting the booze too – not only are you then attempting to keep up a relationship which is based on two insecure people who are not in tune with their own individual needs and emotions, but arguments which arise when under the influence are virtually guaranteed. To make matters worse, dependent drinkers will automatically prioritise alcohol over other people, which can result in selfish behaviour.

Maslow's Hierarchy of Needs model suggests that only

when a sense of belonging has been secured can we progress to establishing self-esteem (achievement, mastery, recognition, and respect). In all honesty I can't recall ever experiencing feelings of mastery and self-respect when I drank alcohol. Occasionally I had a glimmer of a sense of achievement (for instance when I obtained my two degrees) but there was a permanent kernel of self-doubt that obscured any genuine happiness – deep down I always had a hunch that something external to me had enabled me to reach a particular goal; the exam was too easy, I'd only managed to obtain a 2:1 whereas really clever people were awarded first-class degrees, or the 10k race in which I'd beaten my own personal best was run on flat ground and anyone who was reasonably fit could do the same. I never gave myself the pat on the back that, at times, I deserved.

And I was always teetering on the precipice of utter self-hatred. It would take just one comment, the tiniest hint at a particular inadequacy, and I would spin downwards into an incredibly dark place where only alcohol could help relieve the pain. I was far from possessing any true self-esteem when I drank alcohol.

The highest need of Maslow's original model, self-actualization, was so beyond my radar that I doubt I was even aware of the term. This level relates to the fulfilment of a person's potential through having the desire to become all that he or she can. Maslow purported that in order to achieve self-actualization it was essential to *master* the lower-level needs; he felt it wasn't enough to possess self-esteem, but that one must excel in it, have bucket-loads of it, be rolling in the stuff. With the almost non-existent supply of self-esteem I had during my twenties and early thirties, it's hardly a surprise that I remained a long way off effecting self-actualization until after I quit drinking aged thirty-five.

What I have become aware of in the last three and a

half years since I became alcohol-free is that whereas previously I felt as though I had an ongoing hole which cried out to be filled, I now feel content with much less. The old me was attempting to plug a self-esteem-shaped gap in my life with booze, a constant stream of new boyfriends, clothes, and 'stuff' (you know – cushions, candles, jewellery, bags, shoes …), whereas now that my emotional needs are taken care of, that desire to seek happiness from without rather than from within has magically disappeared. Obviously I still enjoy buying nice things – the difference lies in the fact that I no longer feel as though my happiness depends on external factors and if I have to go without, then I can – easily.

I have come to understand that when one attempts to meet an emotional need with 'things' alone, rather than by developing inner contentment, that need will forever remain unanswered. The pair of shoes we buy but can ill afford will not prevent us from wanting another pair just a few days or weeks later; the £25 candle that we know is out of our budget but we feel is a must-have may satisfy the urge for a while but it's not going to work for ever. And the bottle of wine we pick up while doing the supermarket shop because it's Friday night, it's been one hell of a week, and damn, we deserve it, will not be the last one we buy. At least not for as long as we haven't resolved the deep-down issue of rebuilding damaged self-esteem.

Alcohol is a complicated commodity. Because we are trained from an early age to regard it as a sophisticated and grown-up treat, something which helps us to appear glamorous and sexy, just the mere act of purchasing a bottle from the shop can be sufficient to stir feelings of pleasure. Many of the positive associations we create with regards to alcohol lie in the anticipation, the excitement about what we can look forward to just as soon as the cork has been popped.

Once we have the glass in our hand, the booze in our bodies, and the ethanol begins to take effect, the feelings of pleasure are ramped up further. Alcohol *does* induce a false confidence and appears to obliterate all our stresses and worries, and therefore it's easy to focus on these perceived benefits of our favourite tipple. However, when we are devoid of bona fide self-esteem, all we are doing through regular drinking is filling a hole *temporarily*. The feeling will not last and, importantly, when the immediate effects have worn off we will be left feeling worse than we did before. I compare this short-term gratification coupled with worsening an already present condition with biting one's nails. That desire to just nibble off a little snag on your fingertip will not end the compulsion to chew – it will merely increase it, and make the damage caused even more noticeable. Giving into the temptation to have a bottle of wine will not stop the cravings; it will only intensify them and make it more difficult to stop drinking than it was the previous day.

This realisation, when it finally sank in after twenty long years, is what lay behind my success in ditching the wine for good. Wrapping one's head around the notion that *each* drink will only lengthen the battle, increase the cravings, and postpone the resolution of the dependency, is the beginning of escape. In acknowledging this truth and acting on it, the hole that was previously filled with alcohol will suddenly open up – you cannot ignore how unhappy you feel in reality, and this pain can be utilised as a motivating force to repair yourself from within.

Here's what I noticed about myself when I initially stopped drinking: I was bored in the house, I had no confidence in social situations, I didn't like myself very much, and my life was a long way off what I wanted it to be. Alcohol had enabled me to cover up all of these issues which now presented themselves to me in a very obvious manner.

The key to living alcohol-free on a long-term basis is to successfully fill the hole which alcohol leaves behind.

Boredom was a key trigger for me, and so I ensured that I kept occupied in order not to leave myself open to temptation. I had always maintained a semi-commitment to running, even when I was drinking a lot, so I zoned in on that as a pastime to help keep me busy. Any form of exercise is a good distraction in the early days of alcohol-free life as it's a fairly time-consuming business from start to finish – getting changed, warming up, doing the exercise, cooling down, and having a shower takes a good hour or two. In addition, our bodies release endorphins when we exercise which results in a natural high. Exercise is also a good way of eradicating stress (and escaping the house if a bit of solitude and 'me time' is what's required).

My second major hurdle was that I had zero self-confidence in social situations. Making idle chit-chat with an unfamiliar person was an excruciating experience for me; my cheeks blushed, I tripped over my words, and my heart raced. I realised very quickly the extent to which I had been relying on alcohol to buoy me up in such instances, as without booze to lubricate my social skills I was a nervous wreck!

What worked for me in terms of conquering my fear of social interaction minus the prop of ethanol was cognitive behavioural therapy. For six weeks I visited an incredibly helpful counsellor once a week for an hour. He shone a bright light on my emotional weaknesses and provided me with several mental coping strategies to overcome them. I put a lot of work into the tasks he set me and focused hard on my mental state for a good few weeks; it paid off and I soon began to notice that my low self-confidence, so noticeable in the early aftermath of my boozing years, was beginning to grow.

Over the course of a few months, the omission of alcohol together with the time and effort I invested in filling the bottle-shaped hole combined to help improve my life. The ongoing fears that as a drinker had eaten away at me (fear of dying, fear of alcoholism, fear of letting my daughter down) slowly diminished. In Maslow's Hierarchy of Needs model this meant I was free to progress to the next stage – a sense of belonging. The car-crash relationships and poor personal choices made impetuously when drunk or hungover all ceased to exist and I concentrated on just two relationships which were important to me: the one with my daughter, and the one with my fiancé. As this took place, a burgeoning sense of belonging arose – Maslow's precursor to self-esteem. For the first time in my life I felt fully emotionally connected (and emotionally equal) with my partner, and the feelings of guilt, shame, and inadequacy I had often experienced as a result of drinking too much as a parent were no more. This allowed me to enjoy a much stronger bond with my daughter, something which benefited both of us enormously.

Maslow's highest need in his original model, self-actualization, happened without me even registering it, but with hindsight I can see that it occurred after about a year of freedom from alcohol. With every one of the lower needs taken care of I was able to concentrate on becoming the best parent I could be, to develop my creativity, and to establish the social network website Soberistas – these in turn helped to reinforce my self-esteem quite naturally, and therefore the lower needs were safe from unravelling, as they had always done in the past.

While Maslow's model has attracted criticism (for example, that it is ethnocentric), I find it a helpful illustration of how alcohol can undermine our emotional state, making it impossible for us to realise our true potential while ever we are getting drunk on a regular basis. Maslow's Hierarchy of Needs highlights how a sense of belonging, the possession of self-esteem and self-actualization are natural, vital components of a human being's emotional makeup. It highlights how we can prioritize certain aspects of our lives in order to build on the foundations so essential for self-fulfilment.

During the twenty years I spent as a drinker, my self-image altered frequently – sometimes several times in a single day. I often awoke feeling scared and ashamed as the half-memories of the previous night flooded back. As the day wore on I would push those negative emotions to the back of my mind and focus on whatever I was doing, forcing myself to plod on irrespective of the fact that just a few hours earlier I had been blind drunk and engaging in all manner of stupid/regrettable/embarrassing actions. By late afternoon I was planning my next intake of alcohol, and at that point my self-image would switch from a scared shell of a person to a woman who exuded sexiness, confidence, and wit.

There was an inextricable link between the contents of a wine bottle and my ability to feel good about myself. The mere thought of taking that first sip elevated me from a run-of-the-mill, humdrum existence to an exotic, glamorous, and exciting life. Why? How did such a sense of passion and thrill ever emerge from the reality of me under the influence? When I observe drunken people nowadays I see none of the outward signs of sexiness that I witnessed internally when drinking – the flirtatious manner, movie-star sexiness, and entertaining conversations are nowhere to be seen. Rather it's a case of slurred words, slipped features, and loud, obnoxious, and repetitive speech.

Looking back on my transition from child to teenager, I see a pattern emerge throughout school and college. My bolshiness was repeatedly knocked out of me (usually by teachers) and a creative streak that was so apparent as a child was not especially picked up on and developed, resulting in those particular elements of my personality being lost by the wayside somewhere in my mid-teens. Two very core characteristics gradually disappeared, leaving me with a deep-rooted belief that I was flawed and somehow 'bad' as a person. That sense of being no good stayed with me right up until I stopped drinking, when I began working on repairing the damage that booze had wielded on my self-esteem.

Aged seventeen, one of my best friends was murdered, and the knowledge that she was no longer here, while I got to enjoy the rest of my life, impacted severely on me. I felt a massive amount of guilt and my desire to self-harm was ramped up a notch. The notion of being a bad person (which had gathered momentum since my early teens) intensified and I fell into an eating disorder which was to last until I was twenty-three when my first child was born. Simultaneously, destructive relationships with men who I should have stayed well clear of, and heavy, dangerous drinking, became the norm.

And all the way through that very damaging period of my life, which lasted several years, alcohol somehow retained its ability to make me feel good about myself – or so I believed. The initial boozy rush of excitement and giddiness enabled me to temporarily leave the world I inhabited, something which felt pleasant (because my world was not a place I really wanted to be). The false confidence that alcohol brought about enabled me to flirt boldly with men, acting in a sexually precocious fashion that would never have been possible had I been sober. Drinking made me feel on top of the world – in the very short term. The times I spent *not* under the influence during my late teens and early twenties were so few and far between that I gave little thought to the fact that I felt pretty wretched once the effects had worn off. I just kept going back for more. And more.

Despite being entirely unaware during this chapter of my life of the harm I was inflicting on my inner self through the excessive and regular consumption of booze, I was, in actuality, picking away at the meagre amount of self-esteem that I did still possess. Because I was drunk so often I frequently made terrible life choices, which in turn had their own effect on my state of emotional wellbeing. For instance, I didn't concentrate on my first stab at a university degree, instead channelling all my energies into the pub, men, and alcohol. I ploughed headlong into a relationship with a drug dealer (see p.17) who assaulted me mentally and physically, to such a degree that I eventually moved to London to escape his clutches.

Relocating to London consequently meant not finishing my course at Sheffield Hallam University, and scuppering my chances of completing my further education in my early twenties which would have left me free to get stuck into a career. I drifted and, without any real direction, I gravitated towards alcohol for some light relief. My late teens and early twenties were all about getting wasted, one way or another. Every evening I lived in a parallel universe where I thought I was amazingly good fun, the life and soul of the party, and yet which left me so desperately lacking in confidence that I was totally unable to interact with people outside my immediate social circle.

When we surround ourselves with other heavy drinkers, there are significant consequences which make it easy to remain trapped in a boozy existence. People rarely act the same around those they are very familiar with, and those they don't know so well. We gravitate towards friends and partners who have a similar perspective on life as us, and therefore when immersed in a like-minded group there can seem nothing out of the ordinary in day-long drinking sessions or weekends drifting past in a hazy whirlwind of partying and hangovers.

However, once we step outside and interact with people who do *not* drink excessively, it is noticeable just how unsure and lacking in self-belief we truly are. And because those feelings make us feel uncomfortable, we are propelled fairly rapidly back into the land we know and love – the land of booze. As a drinker in my late teens, my nervousness around strangers and unfamiliar situations was so extreme that I virtually experienced a panic attack at the mere thought of having to purchase a train ticket or pay for some groceries at the supermarket. Conversely, self-confidence builds daily in a very organic way in people who do not regularly drink to excess – the reactions we receive from those we interact with helps confirm that we are OK as human beings.

The paranoia I often felt in social situations was created by the amount of alcohol with which I was poisoning my body – but alcohol was the very substance I craved in order to deal with it. Effectively, this was a self-made personal confidence crisis that was to last for twenty years.

Ultimately, if we choose to quit drinking we are selecting long-term contentment (albeit with a temporary rough ride and some painful emotions along the way) over a series of short-term highs and rock-bottom lows. One of the most dangerous outcomes of heavy drinking is that poor self-esteem is often disguised by the artificial feel-good factor of alcohol; it's easy to believe we are self-confident when we focus only on how we act when drinking. However, the bona fide self-esteem which helps push us into going for promotions, embarking on interests where we have to meet new people and challenge ourselves, and striving to attain goals and personal development, is nowhere to be found when we regularly drink excessively. A significant alcohol dependency will ensure a person's potential is capped, and the subsequent lack of achievements in his or her life will reinforce a low self-esteem.

I tolerated this negative cycle because of the association I made at an early age between alcohol and excitement. I gave no consideration to the idea of living without booze because a drinking life was pretty much the only option presented to me – grown-ups drink, and when they drink, it is fun. That message was reinforced all through my life via films, music, advertisements, and by the people around me. I honestly never investigated the possibility of a booze-free lifestyle – there was only one way.

Self-actualization is necessary if we are to gain the tools required for change. In order to understand where we are going wrong, what it is that's keeping us in a place we no longer wish to be, and to work out exactly how to dig deep to alter the particular behaviours that are resulting in negative outcomes, it is vital we know ourselves fully. Being aware of the person inside allows us to highlight all that we are not satisfied with, and, crucially, helps us realise how to improve our lives. Without a high degree of self-esteem and a solid sense of belonging, self-actualization remains out of reach. And without self-actualization, we cannot recognise how we should act in order to obtain different results.

This is the crux of the booze trap, and demonstrates part of the reason why so many people find it difficult to break out of long-standing and destructive habitual drinking patterns.

Heavy alcohol consumption does not make us appear sexy, interesting, or glamorous – in fact the opposite effect is true of all three. Drinking does on occasion, however, (artificially) make us *feel* this way, hence the ongoing attraction. And when we are socialising with other heavy drinkers who all erroneously believe that they are presenting themselves in a similar positive way, it is nigh on impossible to draw the line between fantasy and reality.

Living alcohol-free provides a new perspective. So what if everyone you know still drinks like a fish? Try taking a step back and allowing yourself to be *you*, even if it's only in the short-term. Buy some time to regain a little

of us (Sean, my daughter Isobel, and me). Recovering mentally and physically from my little episode in hospital took up most of my energy, but I found a great deal of pleasure in simply existing free from hangovers and mornings marred by shameful recollections of drunken behaviour. Life felt simple and uncomplicated.

However, as the memories of that awful experience in A&E slowly began to fade, I became aware of a burgeoning sense of unease. I was enjoying my new alcohol-free existence but doubts relating to who I would become as a teetotaller were creeping up on me and threatening my newfound sobriety. As I've said, in my head, Lucy Rocca was a boozer, a rebel, a free thinker – and none of those definitions sat comfortably with the image of a non-drinker, as I pictured such a character in my mind.

Religious people often adhered to abstinence, as did very straight-laced types. People who were not at ease with letting their hair down, and conformists, those who were frightened to live life on the edge; these were my only associations with teetotallers. I felt compelled to discover an alcohol-free identity to which I could relate, and none of the above came anywhere close.

Muslims don't drink alcohol because it is considered sinful to do so. Becoming intoxicated is a sure-fire way of forgetting about Allah (in the Qur'an "Intoxications" are referred to as "abominations of Satan's handiwork"), and this is prohibited. Maintaining a pure mind is essential for ensuring a person's ability to develop their spirituality and move closer to God.

The Protestant Christian denomination of the Seventh-day Adventist Church (as of May 2007, this was the twelfth largest religious body in the world), is centred around '28 Fundamentals', a set of beliefs which the religious movement agrees is vital for living in accordance with God and his will. A particularly healthy bunch of

39

Christians, the Seventh-day Adventists have been found to outlive other Californians by four to ten years (research funded by the U.S. National Institutes of Health), a fact which is attributed to their avoidance of alcohol, tobacco, caffeine, and other harmful substances. A well-balanced vegetarian diet is also advised, as is regular exercise. On the movement's official website there are numerous statements pertaining to all manner of issues such as AIDS, homosexuality, gambling, and booze. It is explained of alcohol and tobacco that, "The Church condemned the use of both as destructive to life, family, and spirituality. She adopted, in practice, a definition of temperance which urged 'total abstinence from that which is injurious, and the careful and judicious use of that which is good.'"[1] With their questionable views on issues such as homosexuality and prescriptions against even meat and gambling, the idea of becoming a non-drinker like this famously teetotal group was a daunting one.

In addition, there was Buddha, who was also opposed to intoxicants of any kind due to their interference with the mind. Meditation as a means of developing self-awareness and achieving a state of true happiness is impossible to practise if one is drinking regularly, and therefore committed Buddhists do not partake in drinking alcohol or the ingestion of other mind-altering drugs. The Five Precepts, the code of ethics followed by Buddhists, includes a reference to abstinence from alcohol (the consumption of which is lumped together with murder):

1. I undertake the training rule to abstain from killing.

2. I undertake the training rule to abstain from taking what is not given.

---

[1] See http://www.adventist.org/information/official-statements/statements/article/go/0/chemical-use-abuse-and-dependency/36/

3. I undertake the training rule to avoid sexual misconduct.

4. I undertake the training rule to abstain from false speech.

5. I undertake the training rule to abstain from fermented drink that causes heedlessness.

Buddhists stress that we cannot obtain happiness via external means; a better job, improved social status, or an expensive pair of shoes will not make us happy because they won't eradicate the many problems and negative events that occur all through our lives. The only way to achieve a lasting sense of happiness is to establish it in our minds – and the way to do this is through a devoted practice of Buddhadarma, or the way of the Buddha. It stands to reason that a devoted practice of anything is impossible when a person is regularly getting smashed on booze.

You may well be asking the question at this juncture: why focus on the above selection of religious beliefs on alcohol? This is why; as the first few weeks of sobriety passed by and spring 2011 gave way to summer's greenness and light, warm evenings, I spent much of my time at a friend's house, speaking to her and her husband about addiction. The husband had in the past been addicted to cocaine, but had not touched any mind-altering substances (including alcohol) in the fifteen years since he entered rehab. My friend (his wife) had never been much of a drinker, but all three of us still maintained longstanding cigarette-smoking habits.

In the evenings when my daughter was with her father (occasions where I would once have been knocking back large glasses of pinot grigio in the stable yard of my local pub), we would all sit in my friends' back garden under a beautiful oak tree, smoking like chimneys and ruminating on addiction, drugs, life, and religion. The husband had conquered his narcotics problem by channelling his love for them into a newfound devotion to God, and we spoke at length of the positive impact Christianity had made upon his life.

I am not religious. On the odd Sunday when I was in my early teens, my sister and I would accompany our grandma to church in rare displays of altruism, and as a child I sang in the local church choir at the weekends (this was one hundred per cent down to the fact it was a paid job; how else does a seven-year-old earn a crust?). Other than those two experiences, and weddings and funerals, I have never given any consideration to setting foot inside a place of worship.

Contemplating sobriety, however, brought the notion of religion to the forefront of my mind. I strongly felt that I needed a replacement to fill the noticeable vacuum that had yawned open in the time since my last alcoholic drink. Perhaps there was, too, a deeper, more subconscious desire to be led by something bigger than I was – a focus that would guide me away from temptation should my resolve to stay dry ever weaken. I craved guidance, and looking back I suspect this was due to a lack of trust in myself; I had, after all, repeatedly made bad decisions throughout my adult life, climaxing in the horrifically bad choice to drink so much that I wound up in a hospital bed covered in my own puke. I had no faith in me and so I was seeking out a better way, a higher being that could show me how to live like a decent human being.

During those evenings I gave consideration to religion in a way that I haven't done before or since. But in the end, I just couldn't scrabble over the boulders of doubt that had consistently stood in the way of me and God since I was old enough to comprehend the whole business of faith. At the time I felt almost saddened by the fact that I couldn't find it in me to follow my friend's example, and my ultimate rejection of any god had the effect of intensifying my loneliness.

It really did just come down to me. Me and booze – many a time it was as though there was nothing else in the world but the two of us.

Spirituality as a means of overcoming an alcohol dependency forms the cornerstone of Alcoholics Anonymous. In the AA's Big Book, it states:

"If, when you honestly want to, you find you cannot quit entirely, or if when drinking, you have little control over the amount you take, you are probably alcoholic. If that be the case, you may be suffering from an illness which only a spiritual experience will conquer."

The first six steps of the Alcoholics Anonymous' twelve are thus:

1.   Came to believe that a Power greater than ourselves could restore us to sanity.

2.   Made a decision to turn our will and our lives over to the care of God as we understood Him.

3.   Made a searching and fearless moral inventory of ourselves.

4.   Admitted to God, to ourselves and to another human being the exact nature of our wrongs.

5.   Were entirely ready to have God remove all these defects of character.

6.   Humbly asked Him to remove our shortcomings.

Now there are many AA followers who will reiterate the point that the Higher Power does not have to be God Himself, but whether a person picks God or a less overtly religious symbol, the end result is the same. The AA functions on the very premise that so naturally worked its way into my thought process in those early days of sobriety; due to a basic lack of trust in my own mental strength, it seemed like a good idea to get behind something more powerful than I was – and to do it fast before I found my way back to the wine aisle of my local Tesco.

However, despite desperate attempts at converting myself, I simply could not find it in me to believe and therefore I continued on the secular path I'd always followed. I began to consider sobriety in a more in-depth way; why was being teetotal so firmly linked to religion for so many people? Why did the issue of faith arise out of my longing to never drink alcohol again? Why, oh why, could I not simply choose to be a non-drinker and just get on with it, free from the need to discover something profound with which to fill that bottle-shaped hole?

These questions continued to whir around my head, and have failed to disappear entirely in the three and a half years since I quit drinking. It is because of a need for answers that I decided to look further into the reasons why it seems that religion, boring people, and teetotalism are so frequently boxed up together, and why I immediately (albeit fleetingly) felt a little bit drawn to God in the aftermath of my last drinking escapade.

I couldn't help noticing a woman nicknamed 'Lemonade Lucy' in my research on the subject of teetotalism through the ages. In fact, I rather fancied adopting this title for myself! Lemonade Lucy, or Lucy Ware Webb Hayes, was married to Rutherford B. Hayes, US president between the years 1877-1881. She graduated from Wesleyan Women's College as a part of the class of 1850 (she was the first US first lady to have graduated from college) and wed Rutherford Hayes in 1852.

Lucy Hayes was heavily influenced by her grandfather in her upbringing, as her father died when she was just two years old. Grandfather Isaac Cook was a fervent advocate of temperance and his views, together with her religious background and the studies she partook in at Wesleyan Female College, Cincinnati, combined to make Lucy primarily focused on moral matters. Her college essays are known to have centred on subjects such as whether society would be correct in prohibiting the manufacture and sale of 'ardent sprits', and world degeneration. As she matured, she developed a growing interest and awareness of women's rights.

Lemonade Lucy was a well-known supporter of the anti-slavery movement, and active in boosting the morale of infantrymen during the Civil War. Her many visits to camp where she engaged in attending the wounded soldiers, comforting the dying, and generally raising the spirits of those on the frontline, earned her another nickname, Mother Lucy.

By the time she entered the White House in 1877, she was well-liked, confident, and, by all accounts, a very popular hostess. She was known for her love of informal parties although this did not prevent her from wholeheartedly backing her husband the president's ban on alcoholic drinks being served at White House functions. By way of demonstrating their approval for this, the Women's Christian Temperance Union commissioned a full-length portrait of Lemonade Lucy which still hangs in the presidential residency today. That being said, Lucy Hayes consistently turned down the opportunity to either lead, or overtly support, the controversial WCTU for fear of politically damaging her husband's reputation.

The nickname Lemonade Lucy did not come about until several years after the first lady's death in 1889. A popular misconception is that it was Lucy Hayes (being the devout Methodist that she was) who initiated the White House ban on alcoholic beverages, and that behind her back employees dubbed her with the moniker of Lemonade Lucy.

However, it is now widely accepted that the first lady was merely supporting her husband's stance on booze, and the couple *jointly* chose to not serve alcohol in the White House because of a number of factors; it was a politically motivated decision, in that it was hoped a dry policy in the president's residence would ensure the temperance advocates in the Republican ranks wouldn't jump ship to join the Prohibition Party; Lucy had always maintained an alcohol-free existence; the couple sought to set a good example and firmly believed that government officials should act with discretion and dignity at all times, something they felt would not be possible if alcohol was on the agenda.

Whether or not her teetotal tag came about posthumously or while she was in residence at the White House, Lucy Hayes was a woman affectionately teased for her alcohol-free views. Certainly it seems to have been more appealing for those who referred to her as Lemonade Lucy to point the finger at her rather than President Rutherford B. Hayes himself for the couple's booze-free policy. There are shades of the lady 'wearing the trousers' in the use of this nickname – as if it is unthinkable for a real man to have come to such a decision as to ban the consumption of booze in his home.

The president's reasons for not serving alcohol at White House functions were, in my view, solid and admirable. However, little seems to have altered in Western society in the (almost) century and a half since Lemonade Lucy was doling out water instead of wine to countless VIPs in attendance at her house. People who choose to not drink alcohol are often subject to suspicion, as if they aren't quite like 'normal folk' who know how to enjoy a proper party.

Alcohol is so engrained in our culture that it has, for many years, flowed freely at dinners, concerts, sporting events, weddings, christenings, birthdays, and Christmases. It is wheeled out as a way of demonstrating that an occasion is considered to be important – after all, isn't a celebration that is centred on lemonade or ginger beer just something for the kids? Alcohol is marketed as a sophisticated and vital component of any grown-up event, and yet when we consider the evidence, this legal drug regularly incites behaviour that is anything but.

I cannot recall a single wedding I've attended during which at least a few of those present were not horribly drunk, a state which led them to acting in an embarrassing or regrettable way (if it wasn't any other guest then you can bet your bottom dollar it was me). At the reception of one wedding, I joined some others for an after-hours party in the bridal suite. Considerable amounts of alcohol were consumed and consequently two of the guests became embroiled in a 'play fight' which climaxed in the hotel's four-poster bed being broken, a black eye, a ripped wedding dress, and a hysterical bride.

I've never been on a Christmas night out with colleagues which didn't conclude with several people being so 'out of it' they couldn't stand, multiple 'sickies' being pulled the following day (as a result of being hungover or out of sheer shame) and one or two members of staff throwing themselves at completely uninterested workmates in a sexual way (I'm guilty of all of these, I hasten to add).

So what is it about alcohol for a vast number of people that, despite its frequently detrimental effect, makes it impossibly difficult to resist, and so much a part of life that its thought to be almost abhorrent to exist without it? And for those who remain deeply in love with drinking, why are people who express doubts over the alleged brilliance of booze often considered boring (at best) and perhaps even excluded (at worst)?

The reasons why I enjoyed drinking so much are, I'm sure, similar to those of most people who regularly consume alcohol. It loosens us up, lubricates social situations, and in doing so it makes us feel relaxed and less concerned with day-to-day worries. When you put it like that, alcohol sounds like a great idea. However, the problems arise out of the fact that alcohol is a drug, and

47

therefore we can become addicted to it – both in an emotional and/or a physical sense. If you had a great time while drinking, letting your hair down and not thinking about the fact that you have no money/are in a bad relationship/are overweight/in a job you hate/are generally unsatisfied with life, why would you then proceed to go out (or stay in) and remain sober? When it's all too easy to obliterate the mundane, the disappointing, and the painful simply by popping a cork, ordering a cold, buttery chardonnay from the wine waiter, or obtaining a chilled pint of continental lager from the bar, why opt for a seemingly difficult evening instead, during which (heaven forbid!) you have to rely solely on the natural, real-life version of you to get through it?

And, if alcohol is recognised as *the* social drug of choice (which it is, across all of Western society, bridging class divides and genders), the few who may decide that this substance does not work well for them and therefore decline to drink it, can be perceived as pariahs and killjoys. Nobody wants their good time quashed by another's sobriety, and no one wants to be told they cannot drink.

For me, this was the crux of the issue; I didn't want to jump ship and join the dry camp. I wanted to remain in my comfort zone and party on with the drinkers, dance with no inhibitions, be sexy and captivating and laugh all night over witty conversations. The stereotype of a non-drinker was so fixed in my mind – it was the religious, socially awkward, boring, straight brigade and I couldn't see how I'd fit in with that way of living at all. And yet by quitting drinking altogether, I struggled to find a way to remain the person I had been for my entire adult life.

I liked Lemonade Lucy's nickname and admired her for her care of soldiers in the Civil War and interest in women's rights, but I wanted to locate a figure in the history books who was both a non-drinker and someone I could really relate to – someone who provided an inspirational example of living booze-free and who challenged my preconceptions about teetotallers being boring, religious do-gooders. And then I discovered two such women; Frances Willard and Lady Henry Somerset.

The temperance movement in the US lost much of its vigour during the Civil War years (1861-65) as interests and resources were temporarily redirected to more pressing matters, but it was revived in its aftermath. In 1869 the Prohibition Party was founded, and four years later, so too was the Woman's Christian Temperance Union (the WCTU who arranged the portrait of Lemonade Lucy, as mentioned above). Together these organisations fought to reinstate interest and support for the dry crusade. The WCTU held firm the belief that alcohol was inherently bad due to the suffering of many women at the hands of their alcoholic husbands. Through education, the group attempted to get the message across to children that sobriety was the way to go – it was hoped that when these youngsters grew up they would transfer that message to the political sphere, thus ensuring Prohibition would be enacted across all American states.

Frances Willard was the second president of the WCTU (between the years of 1879-1898). She was passionate, a force to be reckoned with, and her influences extended as far as the United States Constitution. She played a key role in the Eighteenth and Nineteenth Amendments (Prohibition and Women Suffrage respectively) and zealously encouraged members of the WCTU to be politically active by following her 'Do-Everything' policy. By gaining access to politics via the temperance movement, women were emboldened to challenge politicians on other issues such as prison reform, free school lunches, anti-rape laws, national transportation, and protections against child abuse.

Willard declared that the aims of the organisation were

to create a "union of women from all denominations, for the purpose of educating the young, forming a better public sentiment, reforming the drinking classes, transforming by the power of Divine grace those who are enslaved by alcohol, and removing the dram-shop from our streets by law."[2]

Like Hayes, Willard received a notable education for a woman of her time and after leaving college she subsequently found employment as a teacher. After resigning from her last teaching post in 1874, Willard established the WCTU, becoming active in both the suffrage and temperance movements. Her involvement in the temperance movement was central to her mission (she had witnessed the pain of alcohol misuse first-hand owing to her brother's chronic drinking problems), but Frances Willard was intent on making a number of vast improvements to society, and in particular to the lives of women and children.

She perceived alcohol to be evil, a legalised drug which wreaked havoc on homes and threatened the wellbeing of people all over the world. By campaigning for female emancipation, Frances Willard's desire was to equip women with the means to vote for Prohibition thus affording themselves protection from their alcoholic husbands. She instructed them to abandon the notion that they were the 'weaker' sex, and was forever insistent on politics being a place for women.

Around the same time that Frances Willard was active in America lecturing on and campaigning for suffrage and Prohibition (in 1874 Willard completed a fifty-day long speaking tour, and during a ten-year period averaged 30,000 miles of travel and 400 lectures per year), Lady Henry Somerset was developing an interest in the British

[2] Frances E. Willard, Let Something Good Be Said: Speeches and Writings of Frances E. Willard, Chicago: University of Illinois Press, 2007, p. 78.

temperance movement, partly resulting from the death of her close friend – a woman who had committed suicide while drunk. Deeply religious and privately educated, Lady Somerset was known as Lady Isabel Caroline Somers Cocks prior to her marriage to Lord Henry Somerset in 1872. She went on to become the subject of a national scandal following the birth of her son, Henry Charles Somers Augustus, in 1874, when her husband's homosexuality came to light.

Rather than abiding by the socio-marital convention of the era and maintaining the veneer of a happy home life, Lady Isabel separated from Lord Henry when she finally became aware of his extra-marital affairs. Lord Henry had begun to use the couple's London home as a club where he entertained a close circle of his homosexual friends, one of whom was his wife's cousin. Upon discovery of her husband's activities, Lady Isabel sued him for custody of their young son. The general public lapped up the sordid details eagerly.

In 1878 the courts found in her favour, but the fact that she had refused to maintain the discreet silence that was expected of a woman of her time resulted in her being ostracised by society. She continued to use the title of Lady Henry Somerset and upped sticks to Reigate under a cloud of shame and humiliation. She was just twenty-seven years old.

Isabel experienced something of a divine calling one afternoon while sitting beneath a tree at her home in Reigate. Convinced that she should devote her life to helping others, she proceeded over the following months to reach out to those in need, and in particular became acquainted with the drunken mayhem and poverty which characterised Bye Street in Ledbury, close to Eastnor Castle where she relocated following her father's death. As the locals threw vast quantities of cider down their necks, Isabel recognised that the social degradation in the area was largely as a result of widespread drunkenness. After signing a total abstinence pledge in 1884 at the first meeting of the small temperance movement she set up for her tenants, Isabel established a mission hall in Ledbury as an alternative social venue to the pub. Gradually, more and more were added in the area. Lady Henry Somerset also took on the role of public speaker, delivering passionate orations on alcohol and temperance, later branching out to speak about how a number of social and moral issues affected women.

Isabel did not judge people, perceiving those who fell foul of the charms of alcohol as victims of an addictive substance who needed help and support in escaping its grip. Recognising that people could not be dictated to on the matter of temperance, she expressed the view that no government would succeed in enforcing sobriety but that it could introduce laws which would help people make better choices. Highlighting the economic, health, and social implications of excessive alcohol consumption, Isabel campaigned for 'local option' – a decentralised system which afforded local districts the right to decide whether or not to renew liquor licences. Rather than an outright ban on alcohol, Isabel saw the sense in giving people a choice, something she hoped would empower them and help them achieve self-respect.

In 1889 Lady Somerset stood for election as the president of the British Women's Temperance Association and won. Like its Atlantic cousin, the Women's Christian Temperance Union, the BWTA was primarily opposed to the perceived familial and social disruption caused by male alcohol consumption. Lady Somerset and Frances Willard met for the first time in 1891 and went on to develop a strong friendship. Willard secured the election of her British friend and fellow-visionary as vice-president of the World's Woman's Christian Temperance Association (an organisation of which Frances Willard was president), and the two collaborated often on their shared passion and desire for change until Willard's death in 1898.

To shed further light on the extent of the influence that Lady Isabel Somerset and Frances Willard (et al) wielded on the temperance movement, it is worth mentioning the Polyglot Petition. Written by Willard and circulated to world leaders in the hope that they would take a stand against alcohol and opiate misuse, the petition was signed by an incredible 7,500,000 people in fifty countries. The message of the Polyglot Petition was simple – sober hearts and heads made for happier homes and families, something which governments the world over chose to ignore due to the revenue derived from both the sale of alcohol and opiates. Those who signed were hoping for the total prohibition of these 'curses of civilisation'. However, despite the rather amazing feat of gathering so many signatures in a pre-internet age, the petition did little to bring about any dramatic change.

In 1896, Lady Isabel officially opened the Farm Colony for Inebriate Women, in Duxhurst, Reigate. She was involved at every stage of the creation of this early rehabilitation village, from raising the funds needed to build it, to designing the layout. She also masterminded a number of activities which would serve as alcohol-free distractions for the tenants seeking to overcome addiction.

The Farm Colony was inhabited only by women and children, and had a separate Manor House which was especially created for ladies of a higher social standing, as Isabel believed they were the ones most likely to fall through the net of available help (working-class women had access to other charitable means). Women of all kinds took up residence at Duxhurst, including those who worked as maids, intellectuals, variety hall stars, and even a famous Canadian opera singer. All the women were encouraged to take up community work in the village which Isabel hoped would instil self-confidence and a sense of pride.

A rehab centre that was light years ahead of its time, Isabel wrote of the Farm Colony's 73% success rate in the resolution of the alcohol dependency problems of its tenants over a seven-year period.[3] She spoke passionately and prolifically about drug and alcohol misuse, stating that "... in thousands of cases it [alcohol consumption] is to induce forgetfulness, in others it is to produce exhilaration, in others again it is pure self-indulgence, with the result that the will is impaired, ideals are shattered, and self-control ceases almost to exist."[4]

I was amazed when I happened upon the lives of Lemonade Lucy, Frances Willard, and most of all, of Lady Henry Somerset. Prior to writing this book, I had never heard of any of them, and had a misconception that alcohol addiction services were not created until much later on – and then only by men. For me, aristocratic women of a certain era, their images captured by artists of the time to portray them as very serious and dressed in old-fashioned garments that hang to the ground, strike me as having little gumption and passion for anything other than swanning about with a fan to hand and a gaggle of maids trundling behind them.

And yet Isabel Somerset's devotion to the poverty-stricken residents of Bye Street and subsequently to the hundreds of women and children who stayed at the Farm Colony was outstanding. The speeches she gave which attracted crowds of four thousand and impassioned so many people in the fight against the harms of alcohol stand out as some of the best orations of her time, and yet I had no previous knowledge of her.

Likewise, Frances Willard's efforts in building the

---

[3] Beauty for Ashes, Lady Henry Somerset, Gill, 1913.
[4] A Talent for Humanity, Ros Black, Anthony Rowe Publishing, 2010, p. 99.

temperance movement and encouraging women to challenge politicians on a wide range of feminist matters were wholly impressive. Both Willard and Somerset were motivated by the desire to help people, and especially women who remained a long way from equality in the last decades of the nineteenth century. Their perceptive stance on alcohol, together with Lemonade Lucy's in the White House, was not dissimilar to how I regard alcohol today – it is a substance which, when used in excess, prevents us from acting with dignity and discretion as Lucy Hayes and her husband maintained; it inflames emotions causing tempers to flare and arguments to break out where they may otherwise not have; it's addictive, thus people can irrationally prioritise it and spend money on drinking that might otherwise be utilised more productively; alcohol misuse shatters dreams and results in a loss of self-control.

Once upon a time I would have sneered at a movement so uncool as to be known as the Women's Christian Temperance Union, a bunch of losers who spent their time trying to dampen the good time of total strangers by encouraging total sobriety. Nowadays I am nothing but seriously blown away by what these women achieved (and countless others alongside them).

Even if you take away the religious leanings of Lemonade Lucy, Frances Willard and Isabel Somerset, you are left with three incredibly passionate, intelligent, and proactive women who stood out amongst their contemporaries for their contributions to society at large. Methodists believe that in caring for their fellow human beings through social service they are moving ever closer to God's love. Lucy Hayes and her extensive support of the soldiers in the Civil War, Frances Willard with her impressive fight for a fairer and more equal society, and Lady Isabel who sacrificed so much of her time in running the Farm Colony for Inebriate Women, are, then, all exemplary of Methodism in action.

However, their allegiance to the temperance movement on both sides of the Atlantic could also be perceived as mere common sense, and of being particularly tuned in to the negative consequences of excessive alcohol consumption. Whether religion was a motivating factor or not, I'm somewhat impressed by these women who were brave enough to challenge drunkenness as the norm in an age when female citizens had barely any of the social opportunity that we have today.

For me, long-term sobriety is so intertwined with self-image, the way we define ourselves and our lives, that to remain locked in the headspace we maintained as drinkers amounts to an inevitable return to the bottle. Over a hundred years ago I suspect that the aforementioned women were far less concerned about how their fight against booze reflected on them as people, and that their shared, firm belief that alcohol was a dangerous and socially detrimental substance was something they simply grew up with. They belonged to an age in which most people held religion close to their hearts, and to one in which philanthropy amongst the more affluent was reasonably commonplace.

None of these women had experienced alcohol dependency personally (although Frances Willard's brother and Isabel Somerset's friend both fell foul of the demon drink, which obviously added to their motivation and passion for helping others who were suffering its consequences) and so their efforts to improve society through stricter regulation and/or the prohibition of alcohol were more than likely due to a sense of purpose, rather than as a means of defining themselves.

As the decades have progressed, we humans have become far more concerned with achieving the optimum life. We are overly conscious of how our every decision impacts on personal fulfilment and happiness, and subsequently we stress over where we live, which school to send our children to, how to dress, the diets we follow, the holidays we take, and the exercise regime we try to adhere to; basically, we have more choices than ever before. Even my grandmother's generation when in their twenties, thirties, and forties had nowhere near the number of decisions to make on every aspect of life as that to which we are now accustomed.

When I look back at the way in which my grandmother lived, and how, when compared to me, she was so much more contented with far less, I feel sad at the ways in which modern-day life has spoilt us. While providing a million more opportunities (not least to women), our expectations have risen at an alarming rate and we now want more and want it better than ever before.

The explosion of the media has increased our awareness of how we believe (or rather, are told) we should look and behave. Constantly bombarded by images illustrating the ideal body, face, fashions, and make-up, our lives are under attack from a massive array of competing ideologies and aspirations. And in the midst of all of this we are desperately seeking a way to define who we are, in a way which feels right and natural.

Despite still possessing a profound love for the films and music that shaped my self-image to a substantial degree during my teenage years, it is notable that they were all characterised by a certain level of naughtiness. My favourite film of all time is Martin Scorsese's *Goodfellas* (1990), followed by *Carlito's Way* (1993), and *Scarface* (1983). If you have seen any of these movies you'll be aware that they all follow a Mafia theme, are pretty violent, and depict the less sunny side of life.

I was (and remain) drawn to entertainment that is not pretty. I felt compelled to listen to music that spoke to me about darker emotions and addiction, and to watch films that revealed society at its most violent and anti-authoritarian. Spending my time in pubs as I grew up, around older people who drank heavily and frequently broke the law in one way or another, somehow fitted with the way I perceived myself and my outlook on the world at large. An unconventional and rebellious attitude gradually came to represent the person I believed myself to be – my self-image was formed and alcohol (and the heavy consumption of it) was a vital component of it.

Coincidentally, at the time of writing my mum has just forwarded me the link to an article in today's *Guardian*, entitled 'Which band's beer is top of the hops?' This feature details the rise of band-branded beers, which, as the author states is "… great publicity for the bands, and these beers sell. Last year, Iron Maiden's Trooper turned into the kind of platinum-selling, global smash that made everyone – bands, their managers, and breweries – sit up and take notice. In London, one company, Signature Brew, solely creates ales with musicians."

This is a great idea in terms of commercialism – the alcohol manufacturers are all too aware of the feel-good emotions brought to life by music, and of the associations with 'cool' that so many of us make with our favourite bands and singers. Why not introduce a band-branded beer? They will no doubt sell like hot cakes, and these drinks will appeal to young people more than to any other demographic (catch them young and keep them hooked for life). If I was eighteen years old I would no doubt be first in the queue to buy one.[5]

Fast-forward twenty years to me aged thirty-five, and the old self-image had been manipulated and twisted slightly to accommodate the fact that I was now a parent, had rent and bills to pay, and had a full-time job. But the core strands of my teenage rebellion still lurked and rose to the surface just as soon as I had a drink to hand. The fags, the

---

[5] See http://www.theguardian.com/lifeandstyle/wordofmouth/2014/feb/24/which-band-beer-top-of-the-hops

booze, the endless disastrous relationships, and the derision for all things conventional and proper were still a major part of who I was. I suspected that upon quitting drinking I would struggle to maintain that element of my personality, and I was more than reluctant to let it go. My consideration of religion during the first few weeks I spent alcohol-free was a clear indicator of the need I felt to replace the old me with a new version; I assumed that I could no longer be the 'me' as I had always been, and instead must evolve into a person who might be described as 'a fine, upstanding citizen'. After all, non-drinkers are boring, straight-laced types, right?

The temperance movement figures as described earlier belonged to an entirely different era, one in which people were less self-obsessed and not as overly concerned with how their image came across to others. Facebook and other social media have created a cyber-world in which anyone can become a mini-celebrity – for those with teenage children, the dramatic effect this has had upon their attitude towards aesthetics and the importance of image will be all too obvious. Magazines which dissect the lives and looks of 'celebrities' fill the shelves of supermarkets and newsagents, and this shared obsession with how other people live ultimately impacts on how we perceive ourselves.

Because of the age we inhabit, it is crucial for us as individuals to develop and learn to love a self-image we truly believe in. For me, this has been the absolute reason behind my continued and happy commitment to being a non-drinker – without finding a revised identity by which I am content to define myself, I would most definitely have been tempted to revisit bad habits and old ways.

During the last three and a half years I have upped my feminist leanings, and proudly so. Regular and heavy drinking restricts us, keeps us trapped in bad or unsatisfactory relationships, breeds poor self-esteem, prevents us from reaching our goals, ruins our looks, makes us fat, curtails our ability to create, and then chase, dreams, damages our ability to be a patient and selfless parent, and drains our bank accounts of money which could be spent on more worthwhile things. It destroys our passion and desire to give our time freely to others, it causes and deepens depression and anxiety, and it warps our view of what is important.

Becoming alcohol-free has reawakened my belief that women frequently do not achieve their full potential and that we are often held back in society by a combination of our own low self-esteem, and discrimination. Pouring wine down our necks to anaesthetise ourselves every night only serves to deepen these negative processes by capping all that we are capable of.

Frances Willard, Isabel Somerset, and Lucy Hayes are brilliant examples of women following their hearts and taking action over their beliefs. They demonstrate just what is achievable for those who value society above a bottle of wine and who aren't afraid to challenge the status quo in their fight for a better world. All three have provided me with a fresh way of looking at teetotallers as, despite their religious persuasions, it was their selfless devotion in attempting to save countless lives that really makes these women remarkable.

Although I have no desire to wipe clean my past (at least, not any more – when I originally stopped drinking I would have given a great deal to have been able to erase anything and everything that had made me alcohol-dependent), my perception of what matters has changed irrevocably. Living alcohol-free has made me far more socially conscious and ambitious. I am driven by a desire to work hard and be a good role model for my children; my evenings (some, not all) are spent on writing, working on Soberistas, reading for research purposes, doing chores that mount up during the day when I'm playing with my younger daughter, or helping my older child with her homework. Because of our typically hectic lifestyle, my older daughter and I have ring-fenced Wednesday nights as 'our time' – a sacrosanct few hours when we visit the cinema, do some late-night shopping, or go out for a meal.

I mention the above summary of my evening activities not to appear saint like, but in order to highlight the vast difference between then and now; how in the old days nothing would have come between me and my wine, and the idea of sacrificing a night of drinking to allow me to spend quality time with my daughter would have been unthinkable. Initially I was terrified of living without alcohol because I thought I'd hate the person that sobriety would turn me into. In fact the opposite has happened – I just wish I had taken the plunge and become alcohol-free years earlier.

Chapter Three – The Time is Now

"We all do things we desperately wish we could undo.
Those regrets just become part of who we are, along with
everything else. To spend time trying to change that, well,
it's like chasing clouds."
– Libba Bray

One of the most difficult aspects of adjusting to my new
sober life has been coming to terms with some of my
behaviour during the years I spent drinking.

The self-loathing which arose out of my drunken
actions was a major reason for my continued misuse of
alcohol – rather than face the music I opted to remain in a
state of denial for many years and when I finally sobered
up, I found I had a very bitter pill to swallow. There were
the embarrassing incidents when I'd acted in a loud,
overbearing fashion and the occasions when I'd been
carted off, unconscious, to the spare bedroom at a party.
There was the time on a Christmas night out with
colleagues when I drunkenly swayed across the dance-
floor of nightclub and launched myself (in a 'romantic'
way, not with any violence!) on another staff member who
happened to be almost half my age. These moments,
during which I was acting in a way so far removed from
my true personality it makes me cringe, were bad enough.
But far worse, and a million times more painful in coming
to terms with, was the way in which alcohol affected me as
a parent to my older daughter.

When I discovered I was pregnant aged twenty-three I
stopped drinking immediately. Well, give or take the odd

half a pint of stout – the midwife told me with a wink and a nudge that there was nothing wrong with a glass of Guinness as it was a great way to obtain my iron quota. What's wrong with some dark green leafy vegetables, I ask myself now, but in 1998 that was (and probably still is for many) the accepted wisdom.

So for the eight and a half months following my positive pregnancy test reading, up until Isobel was born in January 1999, I dutifully abided by the antenatal advice supplied and felt great. My desire to drink caffeine and to smoke all but vanished, so cups of tea were replaced with hot water and a slice of lemon, the cigarettes went into the bin, and I enjoyed two-thirds of a year at optimum health. The birth was fairly horrific but after several hours of agonising labour I finally, and delightedly, met my baby girl.

The alcohol remained off limits as I wholeheartedly threw myself into breastfeeding for the first few months of Isobel's life. The same midwife who had suggested I imbibe stout throughout my pregnancy also instructed me to eat a large bar of chocolate with a glass of whole milk every day while lactating. This, she said, would help boost my calcium intake. Eager to do everything correctly, I stuffed my face with a large block of Cadbury's Dairy Milk every night, avoided all other toxins, and happily got on with life as a new mum.

Several weeks later, my (now ex) husband and I decided to venture out for the first time without our new baby and so organised a sitter. Once in the pub with friends I became all too aware of the fact that I had (albeit temporarily) shed my weighty responsibilities for a few hours. After discussing the subject of alcohol consumption during breastfeeding with one of the people we had met up with, I threw caution to the wind and bought a pint of lager. My friend had assured me that her pal, an eminent doctor, was adamant booze could not contaminate the milk supply, and that was that – I jumped back on board the alcohol merry-go-round and was not to dismount again for another twelve years.

Although during the time I breastfed Isobel I wasn't drinking in order to get drunk, I did slowly pick up where I had left off approximately a year earlier before I'd discovered I was pregnant. By the time I switched to formula when she was about four months old I was more than ready to slip back into a shared bottle of wine every night (often with a beer or two beforehand), with a vast increase in my consumption on nights out socialising. As a married mother of one, I was not overly concerned throughout this period about the amount I was drinking. My ex-husband was also fond of a drink, as were all our friends, therefore my penchant for a little glass of something most nights did not strike me as being particularly excessive.

In Isobel's infancy she was a fantastic sleeper and tucked up in bed by seven o'clock most evenings. This meant that her father and I could indulge in a few drinks together without fear of any parenting demands being placed upon us (and thankfully for us, no serious medical or other emergencies arose at any point in Isobel's childhood years). We enjoyed playing the 'sophisticated' grown-ups and frequently delved into the cook books to whip up a fancy meal, always accompanied by expensive wine, of course. The boozing I engaged in back then was seemingly innocuous – mostly we didn't drink until we were hammered, rather we usually had just enough to ensure a little bit of a buzz and a degree of relaxation after a busy day. But, as is the way with the majority of people who consume alcohol on an almost daily basis, there were always the occasions when a couple of glasses weren't sufficient and we drank until we were drunk.

As our marriage reached its close in 2003 there were several instances where the amount I had drunk caused arguments, tears, and recriminations, but for the most part we silently reassured each other that drinking every night was absolutely normal. However, once we had separated and the whiplash effects of divorce kicked in, I hit the self-destruct button and things began to take a turn for the worse.

There are so many reasons why a newly divorced woman will turn to the bottle, and my experiences during this period in my life are largely behind what eventually led me to create Soberistas.com. For a start, I had never lived alone before and was terrified of being the only adult in the house. Drinking helped knock me out at bedtime, and its role as an intended solution for my insomnia was a constant justification for the amount of alcohol I was consuming. I was also seriously heart-broken and somewhat annoyed that my husband of just four years had given me the boot, leaving me to bring up our daughter as a single parent. In addition I was saddled with sole responsibility for the mad puppy we had introduced to our family just a few months earlier.

I was lonely and felt trapped, as once Isobel had fallen asleep I had just the television and the dog for company. I was struggling financially, and also found it hard to navigate my way around the minutiae of life as a singleton; the most basic of tasks such as hanging new curtains, switching to an alternative gas or electricity supplier, or cutting the massive hedge in our garden, were totally novel experiences for me.

But most of all, the impact of divorce left me with a very real sense of being a failure and it is this which caused me to so desperately want to blot out my life by drinking. Very quickly the social, 'fun' element of wine morphed into self-medication – I perceived alcohol as my God-given right, a treat, a sleeping pill, and a mental escape route all rolled into one. Despite drinking on average a bottle of wine a night I still failed to consider my habit to be harmful, other than on the occasional regret-filled morning when things had gone awry the night before and I had consumed more than intended.

In my eyes, wine remained a substance which was middle-class, grown-up, and entirely normal. I drank it in the same way I might ingest anti-depressants or diazepam prescribed by the GP; there was no alternative strategy that I could imagine for getting through that period of my life other than knocking myself out each night, and the socially acceptable nature of wine made it the most obvious choice of mind-altering substance.

The cloud of depression was slowly descending. Despite occasional nights out with friends who all kindly rallied round and attempted to lift me from my misery, I could not shake the overriding sense I had of being a failure. The school playground served as a particularly harsh reminder of all that I had lost; parents of Isobel's friends walking hand-in-hand through the gates to collect their child together, the huddle of happy mums gossiping in the corner, light-heartedly bemoaning their husbands, the apparent lack of anger and bitterness in the demeanour of all those around me – the same anger and bitterness that was eating me alive.

As I stood alone in the playground every afternoon (often as the physical effects of the previous night's heavy drinking began to dissipate at last), my stomach felt knotted and I kept my gaze facing forwards, desperately hoping to avoid any conversations or eye contact. If anyone attempted to draw me into an interaction I would plaster a false smile on my face and do my best to escape the situation; I operated on a wholly 'knuckle down and get out of here as soon as you can' mentality. Every afternoon at 3 p.m. I felt as though I was going into battle.

Later in the evening once Isobel was asleep, out came the wine and I would blot out the pain of yet another day spent living a life I detested.

Just a few months after my husband's departure from the marital home, I began dating. I was driven by a powerful desire to fix my fragmented family, desperately craving a replacement husband and further children in order to have the kind of home life I had always dreamed of. This perhaps wasn't such a bad thing (although I maybe should have waited until my heart had healed sufficiently following the divorce), but what poisoned and twisted my desires into a catalogue of damaging and pointless relationships, was booze.

Because of the social acceptability of not just alcohol but the heavy consumption of it, every dating experience I entered into as a new divorcee was characterised by drunkenness; always mine and frequently the respective man's too. The dates would typically start out with a few drinks in a pub, the second course would be a bottle of wine back at my house (my dating activities all occurred when Isobel was at her dad's), and the dessert a drunken snog (or worse) with talk of future rendezvous – in the pub again, naturally. While all these men were pleasant enough, none of them (and I mean, *none*) are people I would have been remotely interested in had I not been drunk when we first got together.

I have a theory about women and dating (and maybe this applies to men too, but having spoken at length to girlfriends about this matter I *know* for sure it's a common female trait); when engaged in courting, we women are frequently guilty of 'filling in the gaps' with regards to the character of a particular love interest. The parts of the chap's personality which are yet to be unveiled are created in our heads with assumptions of what they might be. I am the world's worst culprit when it comes to this psychological shortcoming, and alcohol, unfortunately, fuels it no end. A little like pouring a bucket of petrol over a barbecue, when a few drinks are thrown into the mix the gulf between reality and fact widens considerably.

Intermittently, during my late twenties/early thirties, I perused the pages of Guardian Soulmates, the dating website for the more discerning, educated, lefty, well, *Guardian* readers, out there looking for love. After browsing the profiles one evening (while guzzling a bottle of wine) I began exchanging messages with a bloke who *seemed* to be all that I was looking for; intelligent, good-looking, not too far away geographically, and reasonably fit (as in the sporty definition, not as in phwwwoooarr). His emails were brief but I didn't worry unduly about this, and even when he explained that he wasn't interested in wasting time to-ing and fro-ing with messages, no major concerns were raised. We set up a date and I looked forward to meeting this man for whom I had very high hopes.

Now, bearing in mind that I knew nothing of substance about this latest romantic interest other than the details of his higher education and a job description, I conjured up a fairly comprehensive vision of him in my head; tall, dark and brooding, somewhat short on words but in a good, Mr Darcy type way, great sense of humour, keen on skiing and running, loved dogs, sensitive and romantic but not in an over-the-top way, a keen fashion sense but not too flashy, enjoyed staying up late into the night ruminating over all sorts of issues with a few bottles of red wine for company … these were all the things I was looking for in a partner. They were not, it transpired, at all representative of the man I met one evening in the pub up the road.

I don't wish to be nasty but my date had all the charisma of a dead fish. We had absolutely nothing in common, no shared interests, and his voice droned on and on like the whirring of a tumble drier. So, what did I do? I drank – a lot. And after an hour or two, him nursing the same pint of weak lager that he'd bought when we first arrived (leaving me to purchase my own drink, and all subsequent ones thereafter) and me on my third large glass of white wine, I magically began to see him somewhat differently. The flat monotone voice evoked an air of mystery, his questionable fashion sense vanished from my radar, and I no longer cared that he was wearing a pair of brand spanking new, glaring white trainers – the type that old people wear for comfort. As the words continued to tumble out of his mouth with all the pizzazz of a damp rag, my addled mind began piecing together his life story until I came to the conclusion that he was indeed Mr Right.

To cut a long story short we went on another couple of dates together (on both occasions I bolstered my confidence with far too much alcohol) until the penny dropped for the pair of us that we were wildly incompatible; I accepted that he was as dull as ditch-water, and he found my excessive love of alcohol to be somewhat problematic and rather unattractive.

This experience was one of many similar 'romantic' adventures, and my unsatisfactory dalliances with the opposite sex gradually became a permanent fixture in my life. With hindsight there are numerous reasons why this period would have been far simpler had it not been for the rocket fuel I was drinking every night; the disastrous relationships with men who were absolutely not right for me would have never begun, thus saving me endless heartache, stress, and time-wasting; my self-esteem would not have taken the extensive and on-going battering that it did as a result of all my regrettable behaviour while under the influence; I would have had much more time to prioritise my little girl and her happiness. However, alcohol fogged up my mind and prevented me from thinking clearly, and I lost sight of what's important.

One of the major effects of drinking for me was that I could not see life as it truly is. What I placed great importance on (i.e. seeking out a second husband) in fact transpired to be of no real importance at all, and I erroneously believed that happiness was to be found externally to me, as opposed to within. I expended vast amounts of energy in chasing dreams, ghosts that I had conjured up in my mind but in reality never existed. I latched onto any excuse or reason which explained away my actions. In particular I remember reading about the love lives of certain celebrities who jumped from one man to the next, often with small children in tow, and I used this information to normalise my own behaviour at the time.

As I introduced different boyfriends to my daughter, and wasted entire weekends drinking while she was staying at her dad's house (always resulting in a dark depression descending on Monday morning which further affected my ability to be a good parent), I continuously managed to convince myself that I was not causing her any harm. It was just modern life, the way people live these days, and because I was a free spirit, unable nor willing to live conventionally. I adopted a false persona as a direct consequence of the amount and frequency of my alcohol consumption, fooling myself into believing that I was in some way enchanting because of the exciting and unpredictable twists and turns my life took.

Alcohol, in fact, suspended my instincts from kicking in. The guilt and intuition which would ordinarily serve to warn me of any wrongdoing simply never appeared. I sincerely believe now that the way I behaved during those years *did* have a negative effect on my daughter, although at the time I was far from able to recognise it.

I lost a degree of emotional attachment to every significant person in my life during the period I spent as a heavy drinker. I prioritised alcohol over all of them, including my daughter. I snapped at her and was unpredictable in my moods – one minute I was the fun-loving mum she could lark about and play the fool with, the next I was biting her head off for no reason, calling time on the light-hearted behaviour and dampening the atmosphere like a sudden thunder cloud descending from a bright blue sky.

There were a handful of instances when I drank so much that I was blatantly drunk and out of control when in charge of my daughter. At my sister's wedding I knocked the wine back all afternoon before my then boyfriend felt it necessary to cart me off upstairs to our hotel bedroom, me shouting abuse at him and falling over. The morning before the ceremony I had spent hours putting together a beautiful outfit, but by 8 p.m. I had mascara-streaked cheeks, muddy heels, and scratches up my arm from where I'd stumbled against a wall outside while smoking. The last thing I remember is Isobel looking at me with a confused look upon her face as I was laid out on the bed in the recovery position, fully clothed.

It's impossible to convey how awful this memory still makes me feel.

There are another couple of occasions which I find physically painful to recall – the night I took Isobel with me to a pub where I was meeting some friends for 'a couple' of drinks, and which culminated hours later in someone having to escort the pair of us home in a taxi because I was not 'with it' enough to get us back safely. The stubbornness of addiction in both of these situations is shocking – how I did not recognise in the first instance that I would never be able to stop after just one or two glasses is something I find remarkable today when I consider the old, drinking version of me. I was consistently without an off switch and therefore it should have been apparent that each and every time I took a sip from the initial drink, I would no longer be able to exercise any control whatsoever.

Alas, this is something which comes with the acceptance that there is an alcohol dependency issue in the first place, and I never did truly acknowledge that until my last night of drinking which landed me in hospital.

The first year I spent sober was jammed full of emotional pain and regrets. The longer I went without any alcohol the more pressing and deep these feelings became. As the booze fog lifted, I developed a far greater understanding of just how highly I had prioritised alcohol and of how irresponsible and downright selfish I had been as a mother. I wanted to crawl out of my skin and sink into the ground to escape the person I had become. I felt such an intense desire to vacate my life and erase all the loathsome actions that at times I felt as if I was losing my mind. You cannot run from yourself, and when alcohol (or any other drug which affects the mind in a similar way) has been removed from the equation, there really is nowhere to hide.

For years I had managed successfully to mentally ameliorate multiple drunken acts of awfulness, simply because of the level of my dependence and the associated denial which is so characteristic of alcohol addiction. I had perpetually reassured myself that there was no real harm being done through my increasing reliance on a bottle or two of wine, continuing apace with getting sloshed without much of a care for anything other than when the next drink was coming my way.

A couple of years after I had my last glass of wine, I contacted an old friend I hadn't been in touch with since my early thirties and who I missed desperately. The termination of our fifteen-year-old friendship had hurt me significantly when it happened initially, but the heartache that arose in the immediate aftermath was nothing compared to the impact that hit me once sober and out of the mists of emotional mutability.

Four years had passed since our last contact, during which time I had smothered the sadness caused by the loss of the friendship and moved on with my life, determined to keep the pain a certain distance from my heart. And yet, as I have come to realise about so many events of my life which I kept submerged with alcohol, the stuff that hurts never really disappears – it is merely redirected to a reservoir of pain, and with sobriety comes the opening of the floodgates and a reawakening of all the searing agony that was anaesthetised initially by drinking.

This particular friend and I first met in that awkward transitional stage of the mid-teens. Immediately drawn to one another in a mutual college class, we became firm friends and would remain so until the age of thirty-three. Simultaneously finding our feet amongst an adolescent minefield of sex, drugs, and rock 'n' roll, we held one another's hand platonically and marched forwards on a shared journey of growing up. He pursued his dream of becoming a musician and I mostly wasted my life on booze, other drugs, and men.

In our early twenties we both forged long-term relationships with other people and naturally drifted apart. Although we kept up intermittent contact we no longer lived in each other's pockets, and met up only occasionally to catch up.

Coincidentally our respective relationships crumbled within a couple of months of one another's, and although it had been approximately five years since we'd spent any substantial length of time together we quickly picked up where we had left off and resumed our friendship. Both then aged twenty-seven, our lives had altered dramatically – I had a child and a mortgage, plus an acrimonious divorce that was to drag me down for well over a year; he shared a rented house with members of his band, had no kids, and plenty of freedom.

Within days we returned to the closeness we had shared years earlier and began to spend much of our spare time together. He was never as enthusiastic about alcohol as I was but put up with my continual desire to drink in the pub, the garden, the living room, wherever, merely out of the fact that we enjoyed one another's company and a tolerance of booze was a prerequisite to spending any time with me.

The loneliness and heartache that we both may otherwise have experienced during this period of our lives was softened considerably by our mutual friendship. The most complicated relationship I have ever known, I was not *in love* with this man but completely loved him and everything about him. The fleeting romances with various significant (and not so significant) others came and went, but he remained a permanent feature on the landscape of my life.

He never approached the subject that I might be an alcoholic; perhaps as he had experienced a family background of alcohol misuse, watching people he loved hurt themselves through drinking was all too normal to him. But no doubt about it, when we were in close contact between the ages of twenty-seven and thirty-three, I had no handle on booze at all and relentlessly drank to hurt myself.

On one occasion we landed late one evening at Manchester Airport following a particularly alcohol-fuelled holiday in Greece, only to race dangerously over the Snake Pass in order for me to be able to buy wine from the off-licence before it shut. I remember starkly the sudden realisation midway between Manchester and Sheffield that I had no alcohol in the house and that, hot on the heels of a wild time abroad (child-free), I couldn't bear the notion of arriving home and simply making my way to bed, sober. We made the shop minutes before its closing and I stocked up on a few bottles as insurance against facing reality.

As our lives meandered along, alcohol occupied an increasingly important part of my world. My existence was characterised by a series of unsuitable partners, the lows of major fall-outs and the highs of reunions, explosions of drunken anger, and introverted, black thoughts brought about my drunkenness – and always a reliance on the bottle to deter the inevitable examination of the truth. A constant source of support and understanding, my best friend remained by my side no matter what, and no matter how little I considered his feelings. In and amongst all the good times we shared, I repeatedly let him down, broke our arrangements at the last minute, and put new boyfriends before him; people who I had known for a matter of days, or even hours.

And ultimately, he grew tired of my habitual lack of regard for him. He walked.

Stubborn and proud, I refused to acknowledge just how much I loved him and revealed none of the bitter pain that now wormed its way around my heart. I drank, as always, to blot things out, and attempted to forget all about him. Two years later I stopped drinking alcohol for good, and gradually, as the sober weeks became months, the number of times during each day that I thought of him and recalled some shared moment we'd had, began to build. I knew all too well that he had been my rock; an unmoving shoulder to lean on with arms that were always there to hold me, an uncanny knack of reading my mind and the ability to make me laugh until I cried.

Over a year sober I bumped into him in the local park and we spoke awkwardly to each other, as unfamiliar work colleagues might address one another out of the office. Unable to accept the finality of the situation I made one last attempt to reach out to him, emailing him a few weeks later with a (no doubt) flippant-sounding, chatty message that concealed the underlying purpose of my contacting him – to make amends and become friends once more, only this time without booze ripping it all apart. His blunt and uninterested reaction was entirely reasonable; he was soon to be married and had moved on, leaving me a long way behind in the wreck of his younger years. I was congratulated for quitting alcohol and reference was made to the fact that, yes, he had always thought of me as a problem drinker.

And that was that, he flitted from my life for ever, a leaf blowing gaily along a path in the opposite direction to me towards a whole new world to which I did not belong.

Losing this friend, my best friend, together with the numerous ways in which I allowed an alcohol dependency to impact negatively on my older daughter's childhood, have been massive in the challenge of letting go of the less-than-rosy past. Initially, I struggled with the idea that we must forgive ourselves for harms done by drinking, for if we are not accountable or punishable for our actions then are we not merely saying it is OK to hurt other people because we choose to drink?

No matter how hard I tried to exercise self-compassion, for a substantial length of time I could not move beyond the fact that Isobel had been frightened by the drunk version of me, her sense of security had been shaken by witnessing me out of control and unable to stand, and her innocent questions had too frequently been met with a hostile, snappy, and unpredicted response purely because I had stayed up late drinking the previous night. I was haunted by memories of my erstwhile best friend laughing with me, the times we had spent together doing nothing but having the most fun in the world, sleeping with each other (but not 'sleeping' with each other), and waking in the morning and cuddling, planning a walk in the countryside, or a crazy last-minute holiday that neither of us could ever afford. I saw his face, full of love, as he watched me land after a 10,000 foot skydive from a tiny aeroplane, I heard his voice telling me that I should start writing; something, anything, just pick up a pen and start …

And I could not forgive myself. I imagined that the rest of my life I would be weighed down by the heavy drag of self-hatred, that the booze might have disappeared but the mess left in its wake was too extensive and ran too deep to ever be cleared away. I would have given so much to be afforded the opportunity to step backwards and rewrite my history. But of course, I couldn't. Nobody can ever do that.

As time has moved on I have grown a little kinder towards myself; with sobriety comes clarity, and with clarity comes acceptance. I perceive the world, and me within it, very differently through alcohol-free eyes, and this alternative perspective has enabled me to draw a line in the sand and leave the past where it belongs. I understand very keenly what it is to feel *regret*; the manner in which it tugs at your heart, how it causes your brain to stretch and contort as it attempts in vain to reach a better outcome. I know the finality of bad endings, and the reality of having to let someone go because it is the best thing for them. I have learnt how painful it is to miss someone every day, knowing you will miss them for the rest of your days.

But I also know of the importance of the present, of the fact that I am still Isobel's mum and I now have the faculties and strength of character to provide her, and her little sister, with the best parenting I can. I accept how strong a hold alcohol once had over me and that it changed me from the inside out, affecting my decisions and behaviour in such an insidious way that I wasn't even aware of it as it occurred. I comfort myself with the knowledge that I am human and we do, after all, make mistakes – all of us.

Three and a half years of sobriety have resulted in a seismic shift occurring in the way I regard myself as an individual. I would love to erase much of the past and alter the course of my personal history in order to protect those who suffered as a result of how I once was, but I have accepted that I cannot. That was then and this is now. I view my life in chapters; the drinking one and the sober one. The person who featured in the old storylines was unaware, blind to reality, and blighted by addiction. Alcohol, in all its potency, wields untold levels of damage to our emotions and thought processes.

And the most startling truth I have come to recognise since quitting drinking is that alcohol muffles life, and all the incredible, beautiful, vital, and remarkable things in it. When we are drinking we fail to notice the intricacies and fragile components of all that is around us. It is too easy when numbing our minds and bodies with ethanol to shut out the deeply significant elements of our relationships, to brush over them with the trivial nature of inebriated conversations and booze-fuelled silliness. The instincts that nature provides us with to ensure we get the job done correctly; the guilt, remorse, and gut feelings that tell us something is wrong, that we need to amend our behaviour, that a partner is not making us happy, that we are unfulfilled in our work, that we are unfit and lethargic when we should be vibrant and bursting with energy and happiness – these early warning signals exist to help us navigate our way successfully through our lives, but they are constricted and warped by the heavy consumption of alcohol.

Put simply, when we drink regularly and to excess, we miss the truth. We do not appreciate that which matters. The intricate web of all that it is to be human is interrupted, manipulated, and tainted. And only when we gain the clarity that living without alcohol brings is a light shone on to the world which reveals it in its true state. Only then do we understand the real extent of the damage our drinking behaviour may have caused.

With an alcohol-free lens on life, emotions are felt properly – something which can take an eternity to grow accustomed to. Feeling pain, happiness, regret, and love to the maximum human capacity is a wholly new phenomenon for a recent ex-drinker and, added to the many changes that are brought about by quitting the booze, this experience of an emotional reawakening can prove hugely challenging. For the first few months of sobriety, my mental state was a constantly changing cycle of highs and lows; one day I was walking on air, the next I was almost suicidal due to the enormity of the multiple regrets that ate away at my insides.

But eventually things settled down, and acceptance became a real concept for me, not merely a word. Despite choosing not to attend Alcoholics Anonymous meetings in my efforts to become a non-drinker, I do find great comfort in the Serenity Prayer adopted by AA and other twelve-step programmes:

'God, grant me the serenity to accept the things I cannot change,
The courage to change the things I can,
And wisdom to know the difference.'

Serenity is indeed what's required to cope with a catalogue of regrets. Over-thinking, blame, self-loathing, and an incessant yearning to unpick events so they can be created afresh are enough to initiate feelings of madness. The mental turmoil stirred up when a person is not accepting of their history can only be quashed with a peace of mind that comes from exercising a degree of self-compassion. We have to understand why we drank as we did, and that when we do consume alcohol excessively and compulsively it prevents us from fully appreciating the harm our behaviour is doing to the people around us.

We need to be courageous to alter deeply embedded characteristics, and to allow ourselves personal growth after years of emotional stagnation, a by-product of heavy drinking. We must be brave in order to accept our faults and undergo a period of transformation where everything feels unusual and strange. It is essential that we cease to fight against what we cannot change if we are to perpetuate a calm and happy mental state which will afford us the strength to stay alcohol-free.

And most importantly, we have to be proactive and positive about the future, and recognise all that we can now offer as non-drinkers, both to ourselves and to those about whom we love and care.

Chapter Four – Sober~~Spontaneity~~

*"You'd be surprised how much fun you can have sober.
When you get the hang of it."*
– James Pinckney Miller

When I drank alcohol I rather fancied myself as being a spontaneous person. I imagine a lot of drinkers think of themselves in this way, that once a glass or two has gone down, inhibitions have shrunk, and the 'fun switch' flicked on, they are transported into carefree mode where they are more inclined to engage in daring or impetuous behaviour.

As previously mentioned, I can recall numerous occasions late at night when upon sinking a bottle or more of wine I'd log on to my computer, fingers would begin to tap away at the keys, and before I knew it I'd be perusing some last-minute city break or other that I could ill afford but that in my sozzled state I talked myself into booking anyway. The people of Barcelona, Budapest, and Sorrento were all graced with my presence as a result of one of these late-night holiday shopping sprees undertaken while under the influence.

In addition I would frequently purchase clothing and items for the home that I simply didn't need or like (when sober), and which were definitely out of budget. As my credit card statement grew more frightening every month, I turned to the only coping strategy I knew of – drinking. And on the merry-go-round would turn.

This impetuousness was something I regarded as a cute characteristic of mine; 'Oh, whoops! I'm so naughty! I just whacked £500 on my credit card again so I can stay in a foreign country for three days – and what's hilarious is that I won't actually be able to remember any of it afterwards due to the whole weekend being lost to drunkenness. But that's me – Mrs Rock n Roll!' Looking back this was all a convoluted manifestation of denial. I was utterly convinced that the elements of my personality which were brought about by booze were part of the real me, that it was my nature to live life on the edge and to be a little bit reckless.

Other examples of this included signing up to a skydive after a few glasses of wine and then doing the jump the morning after a LOT of alcohol had been consumed, a spot of tombstoning (i.e. throwing myself off a large rock and falling rather a long way before hitting the sea) off the north-east coast of Mallorca after a post-lunchtime drinking session, and sending countless emails and texts to recipients (i.e. specifically erstwhile love interests) who I really had no desire to make contact with at all once sober.

However, despite regarding this characteristic as an intrinsic part of me, I was totally convinced that as a non-drinker I would lose this 'exciting' aspect of my personality. Why was this? What led me to imagine that in living free from the alcohol trap I would no longer be able to tap into my spontaneous side?

In his book, *Alcohol Nation* Dr Aric Sigman explains how as teenagers we are physiologically predisposed to behavioural changes which are manifested in '… seeking novelty, taking risks and a decided swing towards peer-based interactions.'[6] . Dr Sigman emphasises that this recklessness is actually nature's way of ensuring the apron strings are well and truly cut, thus prompting us to head out and search for partners not connected to our families,. It also serves to steer us towards leading a fully independent life of our own. But he also points out that this frequently dramatic (and rapid in many cases) shift in

[6] Alcohol Nation, Aric Sigman, Piatkus, 2011, p. 179.

the attitudes of our children can lead to them becoming involved in all manner of endangerment such as '... easy access to drugs, firearms, high-speed cars, boats and motorcycles and, of course, alcohol.' Sigman goes on to state that 'Adolescence is a teetering bridge – a time of great risk and great opportunity.'

I believe this period between childhood and becoming an adult is when spontaneity and booze come to be inextricably linked in the minds of so many people. In teenagers the brain is not yet fully formed, and specifically the prefrontal cortex which controls our ability to plan and to exercise self-control is one of the last parts to mature. This fact provides the biological reasoning behind not only the mood swings of teens, but also their seemingly unquenchable thirst for engaging in risky and daring situations. Our teenage years are also the most common phase in life for developing an initial taste for booze, and excessive alcohol only serves to exacerbate feelings of perpetuity. So intertwined are the natural states of being an adolescent and the false sense of immortality and fearlessness that drinking brings about, it seems almost inevitable that by the time we do reach maturity we are hardwired to connect drinking with risk-taking and excitement.

But let's unpick the consociate relationship between alcohol consumption and recklessness a little more in order to further appreciate how this marriage is realised.

I started drinking in my teens and very quickly arrived at the conclusion that ethanol brought out my 'naughty' side. Even when sober I was usually the joker amongst my group of friends, frequently running into trouble at school for messing about in class and engaging in pranks. Almost certainly borne out of insecurities, I was compelled to act in this fashion by an underlying and strong desire to be liked by all. I enjoyed making people laugh, I relished the sexual attention I began to receive from the opposite sex from a certain age onwards, and I warmed to the reputation I was gaining for my outlandish and rebellious manner. And guess what? Alcohol helped me achieve all of these things – and more.

As teenagers we are champing at the bit to soak up new experiences and to learn as much as possible about the world as a result of our neurochemistry. This is not dissimilar to the way in which nature drives babies and toddlers to thoroughly investigate their surroundings as part of the life-learning curve. If you are a parent to an adolescent, or if you recall your own experiences of youth, you will most likely be aware of the intense passion and motivation that often characterises this age group. Taking part in demonstrations, obsessing over a pop group or film star, or becoming intensely involved in a social cause are all examples of how nature's intention to initiate the learning process manifests itself.

In my mid-teens I wore Dr Marten boots. My hair was bright orange, and I drew kohl in thick lines all around my eyes. My clothes were from charity shops (out of choice, not poverty), my bedroom walls were plastered in floor-to-ceiling posters of The Smiths, The Cure, and Depeche Mode, and I bought joss sticks in bulk. I lusted after boys who smelled of patchouli oil and smoked roll-ups which I kept neatly lined up in a little tin. School was a place where I thought it best to maintain my individualism and autonomy, and I didn't take kindly to instruction or rules of any kind.

I was also extremely passionate about animal welfare, a vegetarian, vehemently opposed to all the repression and prejudice the world had ever known, and wildly anti-fox hunting. I boycotted Boots (the high street chemist) when their penchant for animal testing was revealed in the mass media, and I tagged on to the back of an anti-poll tax march in Sheffield, not particularly understanding what the poll tax actually was. And I hated Margaret Thatcher.

As my personality unfolded during this chapter in my life, so did my attraction towards booze. Because the teenage brain is designed to absorb and retain new information by way of neurological development, it is especially perceptive to habit forming; if an adult takes up a habit, a longer period of time would need to elapse before it became engrained. In a teenager the time frame is much less. In effect, when a younger person begins to smoke or drink alcohol, he or she becomes addicted far more quickly than their adult equivalent would.

To make matters worse, adolescents do not suffer the same degree of noticeable physical consequences (i.e. the severity of hangovers is nowhere near as acute in our younger years) when it comes to alcohol and other addictive substances. In fact, when I was a teenager it was a badge of honour to be so hungover that one vomited – we were proud of how much damage we were inflicting on our bodies!

Therefore, in our younger years we are less likely to care about the harms of alcohol as we first take up the habit of drinking, and because we are of an age when the brain is still being moulded, we are actively hard-wiring ourselves to associate alcohol with fun, recklessness, and all the other 'exciting' elements of the adolescent experience. Add to this the sociological and cultural representations of alcohol that people grow up surrounded by, and it's no great surprise that a tenacious bond connecting drinking with 'letting our hair down' and being spontaneous is formed by the time we reach adulthood.

What, then, is the exact meaning of 'spontaneous'? The Oxford Concise English Dictionary provides the following definition; "performed or occurring as a result of an unpremeditated inner impulse and without external stimulus." The spontaneity that I imagined I was engaging in at any point in my drinking life did not fit with this meaning at all. Rather it could be described as "recklessness and stupidity arising out of a deep-rooted sense of low self-worth and a burning desire to fill a gaping hole, a hole which I had no knowledge even existed prior to becoming alcohol-free".

Certainly the caveat that to be spontaneous one must not be motivated by any 'external stimuli' would make the behaviour of any heavy boozer categorically unspontaneous.

One of Google's earliest engineers, Chade-Meng Tan, once said, "If the mind is calm, your spontaneity and honest thoughts appear. You become more spontaneous." (This man's official job title incidentally is Google's 'Jolly Good Fellow' and he really knows his stuff when it comes to human happiness.) Tan also maintains that "Habits are highly trainable. And habits become character."

When we are not being spontaneous, we are planning, ensuring we have covered all bases, and playing out entire scenarios in our minds before committing to putting anything into practice. Sometimes we can become paralysed by anxieties and fear over the potential consequences of our actions and this prevents us from beginning a particular venture altogether. Contrary to the way I once considered myself as a person (i.e. spontaneous, live life for the moment), as a drinker I engaged in an awful lot of planning and very little spontaneity.

When I drank, alcohol was of the utmost importance to me – I would never have entertained the idea, for instance, of hopping off for a last-minute weekend jaunt to stay with friends in the country or a mini-break in Europe, had there not been booze on the agenda and lots of it. Nights out took a fair degree of planning owing to the fact that I wouldn't sacrifice my alcohol intake for the sake of having easily accessible transport, i.e. my own car. Taxis, a lift or, my particular favourite, drive to the venue but leave the car there until morning when I would jog down to reclaim it, were all preferable alternatives to driving and having an alcohol-free night. The latter option had the double advantage of helping to reinforce my erroneous belief that I didn't have a drink problem (I can't do, I can run five miles with a hangover!)

For any addict, careful planning is an integral part of daily life. It's vital to ensure that one's supply won't run dry, particularly if the availability of additional booze is restricted for whatever reason (Christmas opening hours, for instance). How about if one of the guests coming for dinner is an excessively heavy drinker? Better double up on bottles just in case – hell, it will all get drunk at some point, if not tonight. What if a night's boozing has to be curtailed (for example, if one is socialising with people who don't drink much at all) – just to be sure of obtaining the requisite amount, it might be wise to stock up on a few bottles for when you can escape their company and get home to a proper drink.

The mind of the addict is forever plotting and exercising caution, covering all bases, and making damn sure the booze cabinet is never emptied.

From an early age I taught myself how *not* to be spontaneous by slipping into the habit of regular drinking instead. As a teenager I would hurry home from school on a Friday afternoon, desperate for the end-of-week rituals which began with watching *Neighbours* on the television, a cup of tea and final phone calls to firm up the evening's entertainment, and ended with me blind drunk somewhere in my hometown of Sheffield. My friends and I would always frequent the same pub, where week on week I would drink one of two beverages (bottles of K, the 'designer' cider, or pints of Lowenbrau, both of which were *de rigueur* in the early 1990s, and the nights would always conclude with the same levels of debauchery and drunkenness.

As I grew older, my choice of drinks, venues, and

friends all changed but the heavy boozing remained, as did the rituals which were always attached to it.

Within the constraints of heavy drinking, I did engage in what one might term 'spontaneous behaviour'; that is to say that I might have suddenly thrown a drink over someone's head who had said something which annoyed me, or decided on a whim to accompany a bloke I'd had my (inebriated) eye on back to his pad. But these were not examples of positive spontaneity – they were instances where all the worst elements of my personality came to the fore due to the amount of alcohol I had consumed. The pint-throwing only happened twice but both times I was out-of-control drunk and attempting to assert myself when faced with a person by whom I felt threatened.

The external stimuli which, according to the Oxford English Dictionary, negate a situation having the characteristic of being 'spontaneous', were very much present; I was drunk, angry, showing off, and more than likely hoping to impress people nearby. Late-night rendezvous with men I hardly knew are examples of past behaviour that I'm not especially proud of, and such instances certainly failed to constitute any spontaneity on my part; rather they merely provide further evidence of how little I once valued myself.

Taking into consideration that during my drinking days I repeated the same mistakes over and over again and lived an incredibly restricted existence which revolved around the same people, pubs, and behaviours, it's a wonder how I ever came to the conclusion that I could have been described as 'spontaneous'. Cultural influences must be held accountable in part for providing us with the notion that getting drunk is a free-spirited activity prone to bringing about crazy and fun times.

Off the top of my head I recall Rizzo in the film *Grease* – the cool, rebellious leader of the Pink Ladies who breaks open a bottle of booze and asks 'How about a little sneaky

Pete to get the party going?' at Frenchy's sleepover. Exuding confidence and an adult awareness which is lacking in her peers, Rizzo's use of alcohol in the scene is portrayed as exciting and somewhat naughty. I think of Donna Sheridan and her friends in *Mamma Mia*, a film which is a riot of spontaneity and living for the moment, sharing a bottle of champagne early in the morning and becoming all giggly as they throw caution to the wind and forget about their responsibilities for a while.

Whether we are conditioned through the mass media to believe that alcohol transforms us into more exciting people, or if we all come to that conclusion alone, is something of a chicken and egg situation. It would be unrealistic and nonsensical to point the finger of blame at any one of these films, or the thousands of others like them which promote excessive alcohol consumption as being cool. Nonetheless, the extent to which my drinking behaviour (and therefore no doubt plenty of others') was affected by popular culture's representation of booze was huge. Drinking and getting drunk has, for years, consistently been portrayed as something which cool, edgy people engage in, in films, advertising, music, and books. Such cultural influences, however, rarely highlight a person with a supposed 'drinking problem' as the hero or heroine of the piece, because we, as a society, do not regard such an affliction to be aspirational.

Drinking alcohol is routinely presented as being sophisticated, grown-up, rebellious, fun, off the wall, naughty, sexy, spontaneous, social, and convivial. By the time we reach adulthood, is it at all surprising that we then come to associate a bottle of wine with all of these positive characteristics and more? Is it any wonder that when we drink, we too imagine that we will suddenly possess all of these features?

But if spontaneity is impossible to achieve when we are encumbered by external stimuli (i.e. the effects of alcohol which impinge on our ability to genuinely act in a free-spirited fashion), can we be spontaneous when we are alcohol-free? And why do so many people who are on the cusp of quitting drinking fear that as a non-drinker their lives will become less extemporaneous?

In order to allow spontaneous thoughts to spring to life it is necessary to possess a relaxed mind, devoid of anxieties and stress. It has taken me a very long time (and it's a work in progress but I'm getting there) to learn how to relax properly without any false props or accelerators but simply through the power of the mind. Meditation has helped tremendously with this realisation. When I manage to pull it all together and reach that mental oasis, where the brain ceases to whir at a hundred miles an hour and I experience utter calm from my head down to my toes, that's when I know I'll be thinking up new ideas imminently.

If you are bogged down with mental clutter then there is no room for new thoughts, and certainly not for positive or inspirational ones.

When I was newly sober I spent several months where I seemed to retreat into myself. I felt almost agoraphobic at times and was terrified of letting go of my imagined safety net. Drinking on an almost daily basis and to excess for many years, I had unknowingly thwarted my personal growth and the extent to which I explored the world around me. I had ultimately become a medium-sized fish in a small pond; in my immediate surroundings and with the people I felt familiar with (and of course with a glass of wine to hand), I came across as confident and good fun, someone who engaged in spur of the moment bouts of silliness without caring what anyone thought.

But as soon as I embarked upon an alcohol-free lifestyle I was all too aware of how small I felt, and how frightened I was to let go and just *live*. As if I was marooned on an island in the middle of a shark-infested sea, it was far too scary to take even one step in any direction. I was paralysed with fear over letting myself become *me* again, and it was approximately a whole year before I felt brave enough to test the murky waters that surrounded me.

Alcohol acts in two ways which can cause us to feel nervous in certain social situations and of dipping a toe into the unknown. Firstly, as alcohol-dependent people we habitually prioritise drinking above most other factors in our lives; it becomes engrained in our daily existence to plan around the imbibing of booze. Down to the tiniest detail we are masters in the art of alcohol consumption and this leaves no time to be spontaneous because we are essentially prisoners of the bottle. For decades, in many cases, we are so accustomed to *not* living for the moment, of never being able to drop everything and just do something wildly out of character, that when we do eventually become alcohol-free it can take a while before we are able to alter old habits and think more freely.

Secondly, as heavy drinkers we often act in ways which are stupid, embarrassing, shameful, and regrettable. As far as my own drinking history goes, the mornings, days, and entire weekends lost to self-loathing are too numerous to recall, and all of this negativity made a gradual but ultimately colossal dent in my self-belief. I stopped depending on my instincts many years ago, and to reclaim that trust in myself has taken a substantial amount of time.

In order to be truly spontaneous it is essential to a) be free from worries and anxieties and b) to like and trust yourself sufficiently to allow the mind to go into freefall. For heavy drinkers, both of these states are impossible to achieve.

It is surprisingly easy to avoid new situations and challenges when we initially quit drinking alcohol, thus the opportunity to learn a new way of life is lost. Hiding away from the world (as I tried to do in the early phase of my sobriety) may feel like the safe option but all that it achieves is to reinforce the erroneous belief that alcohol equals fun, and sober equals dull, and it prevents one's character from growing. Yes it does feel scary in the beginning to enter into new situations when sober, but doing so really speeds up the time it takes to work out that life without booze can actually be (despite popular opinion) much more fun!

For me, as an innately shy person who relied on alcohol as not only a crutch when socialising, but as an entire set of limbs, it was something of an uphill struggle to force myself into living rather than to remain at my default setting of hiding. But with every new experience conquered as a sober person, my confidence and trust in myself, and in other people, has grown exponentially. And as my confidence has increased I've rediscovered the ability to be spontaneous. Nowadays I might have a totally out of the blue thought but I presume it will be a good one; I act on it and it usually works out fine. At the very worst I might not end up with the outcome I was hoping for, but there sure as hell won't be any of the alcoholic fallout of days gone by, when a blast of spontaneity was likely to result in anything from a seriously hammered credit card to waking up in bed with someone whom I didn't even like very much.

When I spend time with my toddler and observe her mind jumping freely from one thought to the next, it's clear to see how as children we don't (usually) suffer the encumbrance of any anxieties or fear. Being free-spirited means reconnecting with our inner child; it allows us to let go (temporarily) of any ideas of conventionality in order to do something out of the ordinary. However spontaneity is realised, when our lives (and thus our minds) don't revolve around alcohol such behaviour is enjoyable and provides us with a positive break from the norm.

As Franklin D. Roosevelt famously said during his

inaugural address in 1933, "So, first of all, let me assert my firm belief that the only thing we have to fear is ... fear itself – nameless, unreasoning, unjustified terror which paralyzes needed efforts to convert retreat into advance." Assert to yourself that in the aftermath of the fight against booze there is a real need to transform irrational fears into an advance upon the world. And remember with each act of spontaneity, it becomes easier to do – just as Google's Jolly Good Fellow Chade-Meng Tan said, habits are trainable. It *is* possible to rewire the brain to think differently, and to break long-term behavioural patterns.

So what can you expect to gain by acting in a spontaneous manner in a newly alcohol-free life? Spontaneity forces us to live in the present moment; it goes hand in hand with mindfulness. This is crucial if we are to forget the mistakes of the past, learn how to trust ourselves again, and remain grateful for the things around us (which serves to reinforce a commitment to sobriety). Challenging ourselves to try out new (and perhaps scary) experiences helps us to realise that anything is possible, boundaries are often only imagined, and the world can be our oyster if we choose to break out of the constraints of fear and low self-confidence.

Acting in a free-spirited way also helps us to feel properly alive and energised – the world keeps on refreshing itself over and over again. Life becomes more as we remember it from childhood, where every situation was novel and exciting and each day provided a massive learning curve. Living in a spontaneous way once we are free from the alcohol trap really helps us to trust ourselves again. It speeds up the mental recovery process after years spent living within the restrictive self-imposed boundaries that are so frequently the norm for heavy drinkers.

And most importantly of all, being spontaneous brings about masses of guilt-free fun for non-drinkers. Gone are the terrible consequences of misguided, reckless drunkenness so often mistaken for spontaneity; instead we can enjoy living life for the moment, pushing ourselves to try out new things on a regular basis, and rebuilding the trust in our instincts that we lost so long ago through alcohol dependency.

There's no better time to get into the habit of spontaneity than right now!

Chapter Five – Ladies' Night

"Above all, be the heroine of your life, not the victim."
– Nora Ephron

A study published in the British Medical Journal in 2013 highlighted a worrying trend in the number of alcohol-related deaths amongst women born in the 1970s. Women in this cohort across the three cities examined in the study, Glasgow, Manchester, and Liverpool, experienced disproportionate increases in alcohol-related mortality. The researchers who conducted the study stated that it was "… imperative this early warning sign be acted upon if we are to reduce the number of UK deaths caused by drinking in the long term".

The women in this cohort all grew up against a background of similar childhood environments and cultural messages present at the age when they were first introduced to alcohol. I am one of these women, born slap bang in the middle of the 1970s – October 14th 1975. When the study's findings were published in July 2013 I was invited on to the BBC's *Breakfast* programme alongside one of the researchers behind the study, Deborah Shipton, to provide a personal perspective on how being born in this era had shaped my own predilection to alcohol misuse.

On the programme I discussed the two factors which I believe most shaped my relationship with alcohol (in addition to any specific physiological or psychological characteristics I may have that possibly predetermine an addictive mind set); the 'ladette' culture of the early-mid

1990's, and the powerful and effective marketing strategies employed by wine manufacturers that have unfolded over the last twenty years.

Out of the feminist uprising of the late 1960s and 1970s emerged several socio-cultural trends and events which quite probably contributed to the birth of the 'ladette' in the early 1990s. Growing up in the suburbs of Sheffield, South Yorkshire, my parents were both big believers in gender equality and, rightly and passionately, brought my sister and me up with the opinion that there should be no obstacles in life which exist simply because one is female. In the late 1970s and early 1980s in middle-class middle England it seemed that the vast majority of my friends' mothers, if not both parents, were of similar feminist mindsets.

Our mothers were, for the most part, strong, liberal, independent types who had careers and lives outside of their husbands and families. This was the age when the female juggling act came to be recognised as standard – the majority of my friends and I had mums who were constantly switching hats between that of home-maker, worker and parent, rushing home to begin preparing dinner after a long day at the office (or classroom in the case of my own mother who was a secondary school teacher). This generation of women were the first to be referred to as 'having it all', and their children, me being one of them, were frequently brought up to accept this multi-tasking business as the norm. I never questioned for a minute whether I would attend university and proceed to have a career, nor did I doubt that one day I would have a family of my own.

In *Drink, The Intimate Relationship Between Women and Alcohol* Ann Dowsett Johnston asks of her and my mother's generation, 'Did we have it all? With courage, endless creativity, and gusto, we certainly tried. Without a blueprint, many of us established excellent careers while raising children and nurturing marriages, juggling deadlines, child care, and housework. We experimented with full-time, part-time, flexitime, and freelance work, nannies, day care and shared babysitters, home offices and virtual offices'.[7]

My mum (who undertook an MA at a period in her life when she had two teenage daughters and a full-time teaching job all placing heavy demands on her) and her friends did such a good job of 'having it all', however, that it never occurred to me that it might be bloody hard work.

In the 1970s and 1980s children had infinitely more freedom than that which most are granted today. My childhood home was located on a cul-de-sac almost exclusively inhabited by families, and my friends and I whiled away our weekends and evenings roller-skating and cycling up and down the road, playing in the nearby fields and woodland, and flitting in and out of one another's houses without a care in the world. We learnt via this gay and carefree time a great deal of self-reliance. By the age of twelve I was infinitely wiser in the ways of the world than my older daughter would grow to be at the same age. The safeguards that seem so commonplace today did not exist (at least to nowhere near the same extent) thirty years ago.

As a small child my immediate world felt secure and friendly although I was vaguely aware of a general mood of resilience against authority represented in the popular culture of the day. I intrinsically understood the value of questioning the world around me. My best friend's mum hot-footed it to the Greenham Common Peace Camp on more than the odd occasion to join in the protests for nuclear disarmament. The same friend and I wore our pro-miner's badges with pride during the miner's strike of 1984-5. Virtually everyone I knew was vehemently anti-

---

[7] Drink, The Intimate Relationship Between Women and Alcohol, Ann Dowsett Johnston, Fourth Estate, 2013, p. 44.

Thatcher.

Live Aid in 1985 when I was ten years old was a musical manifestation of the active 'people power' that seemed so characteristic of the age. Bob Geldof in his fight to force Western society at large to stand up and take notice of the famine in Ethiopia, brought together impassioned pop heroes of the time – Queen, U2, David Bowie, Paul McCartney, Elvis Costello – who, to me as a little girl, seemed to take over the world momentarily.

A few years later, stirrings of liberalisation in the Eastern Bloc led to East Germans being allowed to visit West Germany for the first time in decades. Images of celebrations and emotional reunions appeared on the news as people began to cross the wall, climb upon it, and chip away pieces of its brickwork as souvenirs, and I remember a general sense of euphoria and wonderment as this monumental political event worked its way to a crescendo with the eventual fall of the Berlin Wall in 1990.

Towards the end of the same year, when I was in my mid-teens, Margaret Thatcher was forced to stand down as prime minister. On that November day in Sheffield, a city particularly devastated by over a decade of Tory governance, complete strangers were hugging each other in the street, people walked around with big smiles on their faces, and there was an overall feeling of revolution and excitement at what might be around the Thatcher-less corner. As an ardent supporter of the left and a teenager with an air of rebellion about me, I wholeheartedly joined in the celebrations and enjoyed a real taste of political history in the making.

Music in the late 1980s/early 1990s era was dominated by the influence of 'Madchester'; the Happy Mondays, Stone Roses, Inspiral Carpets and the Charlatans had all picked up the baton from bands such as The Smiths, Joy Division, and New Order and were dictating an entire subculture defined by their flared trousers, bowl haircuts, and passion for ingesting excessive amounts of recreational drugs. This was the period in which I first discovered marijuana, and when I dipped a somewhat wayward toe into the underground rave scene. The political background that I and my peers had entered our teenage years against was instrumental in the growth of the new rave culture. There was an air of revolution, talk of 'reclaiming the streets' and a disregard for rules – especially those laid down by the police – but it should be stressed that all of this occurred under a canopy of non-violence, a modern-day peace and love mentality that was similarly all the rage back in the 1960s.

At the weekends nightclubbing frequently led to attending illegal raves in warehouses or out in the countryside a few miles from where I lived. When the clubs closed for the night, convoys of cars would snake up through the city streets and out to darkened moorland and fields where an illicit gathering would be waiting, thumping music and pulsing lights filling the sky. For the next three or four years I was heavily involved in this scene and very rarely witnessed any of the carnage that was, and remains so much a part of drunken Saturday nights out in city centres. An unspoken and assumed love of anyone and everyone who belonged within the rave subculture meant that hugging and kissing complete strangers was a million times more likely than fighting or arguing.

The friendship groups that I was a part of during this period were notable for their egalitarian nature. Lacking the more traditional division of male and female tribes, we mingled together on an even playing field and when we weren't dancing until the early hours with each other, we were drinking pints and playing pool in the local pub. Life seemed to be about having a good time above everything else, and the people I socialised with stemmed from all walks of life, classes, and educations. A shared love of dance music and 'free love' ideals bound us together as, what felt like, members of a secret club.

Gradually the rave scene grew more mainstream and the illegal parties all but ceased to exist. Not long after this I scaled down my affections for recreational drugs and rekindled the flame with my old love, alcohol. By the time I reached my late teens the 'ladette' had most definitely made her presence known on the cultural landscape. Zoe Ball and her best mate Sara Cox were often snapped by the paparazzi swigging pints and 'larging it' in Ibiza with bravado and nonchalance. Perhaps unfairly (and Zoe Ball is notably now a non-drinker, as is her husband Norman 'Fatboy Slim' Cook) Ball and Cox came to represent the 'ladette' figure, and the British media latched on to their antics, together with figures involved in the Britpop scene, with voyeuristic enthusiasm.

My female friends at university mostly fell within the realm of the ladette and we all had similar political, social, and economic values. My personal experience of this social phenomenon was predominantly one of equality; we weren't outlandishly feminist in that we retained our femininity, but we wanted, expected, and (usually) obtained parity with the boys. It seemed to be a matter of *rights*, of fairness and how we envisaged the world should be. Gone was the old-fashioned notion of a lady's glass, and nightclubs that continued to advertise 'Ladies' Night' appeared archaic and downright sexist. I would have been appalled if I'd been bought a half a lager in a delicately-styled glass, and opted instead for pints of frothy Boddingtons.

Being a ladette was about having balls. This bolshiness was a result of growing up that way rather than it being a conscious choice; we weren't wrapped in cotton wool as kids or young teenagers, and we had been raised by parents who didn't follow the stereotypical, by now slightly old-fashioned model of homemaker mum and breadwinner father. Women had enjoyed economic independence for a substantial number of years and the adage of 'she can have it all' was, by the 1990s, so ingrained into Western society that it would have been totally unthinkable to consider stepping back into a lifestyle more typical of the post-war era.

Alcohol, for me and the group of friends with whom I socialised, was merely another element of the Western lifestyle in which we deserved to indulge in equal measures as our male counterparts – and why not? We had the same in pretty much everything else and therefore it would have seemed strange if we had not consumed alcohol with equal fervour. 'Cigarettes and Alcohol' – virtually an entire generation was summarised in the Oasis song that played on pub jukeboxes up and down the country, and there was not a great deal separating the boys from the girls.

To a substantial degree the years I had spent partying amidst the rave scene conditioned me to drinking vaster quantities of alcohol than I might otherwise have done, and to worry little, if at all about the health consequences of doing so. I had observed hundreds if not thousands of people at raves who were overtly out of it on drugs. It was a common occurrence to trip up over the bodies of passed-out clubbers lying in the corner of a nightclub 'chill-out' room, the ecstasy they'd swallowed having temporarily knocked them out. Attempting to begin a conversation with someone on the dance floor only to discover he or she was inhabiting a parallel LSD universe and thus had absolutely no idea where they were or what was going on around them, was entirely normal. By the time I turned my back on drugs, alcohol appeared to be completely harmless – a mind-altering substance for when you stopped taking the *truly* mind-altering substances.

A typical weekend of this period in my life would include a Friday night of reasonably heavy drinking in the pub with a few games of pool, followed by a gathering back at someone's house where we'd listen to music and smoke joints until the early hours of Saturday. The next day would be one long build-up to the highlight of the week: the nightclub or booming house party that we'd been looking forward to since the previous Saturday. Emotional and hungover, our Sundays would be characterised by a mammoth drinking session beginning at 11:30 a.m. when the doors of the pub opened, and terminating at 11 p.m. when we were thrown out.

At that time all the people I associated with, as well as myself, seemed disenchanted with the world at large. We existed within a micro-bubble of alcohol and drugs, only ever socialising with other hedonistic types who could be described as modern-day hippies. I was a student at Sheffield Hallam University and put a certain amount of effort into my studies, but I had absolutely no career aspirations to speak of and viewed the future as a never-ending party. Some of my older friends had already begun their working lives, the weekends of drinking and mayhem impacting on their ability to apply themselves properly Monday to Friday. Several would report that they'd spent much of Monday and Tuesday hiding in the office toilet, unable to hold a conversation with anyone or tackle their workload due to the severity of their hangovers.

A uniting factor of virtually everyone I knew back then was the absolute prioritising of drinking and the party life over everything else. Why were we like this, to such an extreme? My immediate circle of friends had all achieved reasonably good grades at school, and each had a substantial number of qualifications up to (or part way to attaining) university degree level. We were all raised in loving homes, our parents were responsible, and we had never particularly wanted for anything. In Dominic Cavallo's book, *A Fiction of the Past*, the author outlines psychologist Kenneth Keniston's suggestion that children raised in the sixties in America possessed a 'sense of specialness' due to a permissive approach in their upbringing. I wonder if this too had an effect upon children brought up during the 1970s and 1980s as the offspring of liberal, middle-class parents. My own mum and dad consistently treated my sister and me as equal individuals with opinions that counted, from a very early age. We were never brushed away with the Victorian attitude that children should be seen and not heard. Did this ultimately result in a sense of being untouchable, that we were ring-fenced from disaster no matter what we did or said? That the choices we made in our teens and early twenties were valid and acceptable, even if they were questionable at times?

I grew up with a real sense of being free to live my life exactly how I chose, and didn't feel especially compelled to strive for a glittering career. I assumed I would attend university but had no concrete plans for post-graduation. And yet in my late teens/early twenties I did not characterise myself as a loser, rather it felt rebellious and freeing to devote my energies to the good life as opposed to sweating over job interviews and rapid promotions. As a woman, who in times gone by may have been subjected to societal pressures to act in a more reserved and feminine manner, I did exactly as I pleased and found a tribe of similarly-minded individuals who reinforced my somewhat laissez-faire ideals.

I was cocky and unbothered by life outside my social circle. Reminiscent of the girl in Pulp's hit of 1995, 'Common People', I willingly rejected my suburban routes and opted instead for a life of drinking, smoking Marlboro Lights and hanging around pool tables in pubs – 'Smoke some fags and play some pool, pretend you never went to school'. I looked to female idols of the time, the supermodel Kate Moss, DJ Sara Cox, Justine Frischmann of Elastica, the artist Tracey Emin, and girl band All Saints for inspiration and reassurance that this life of necking pints of lager and partying hard was OK and the thing to do in the mid-1990s.

My musical tastes predominantly focused on Oasis, Blur, Pulp, The Verve, and the Manic Street Preachers. Films that inspired and which I could relate to included *Basic Instinct*, *Trainspotting*, *True Romance*, *The Usual Suspects*, and *From Dusk Till Dawn*. Popular culture provided sufficient evidence that there was nothing wrong with living a life of hedonism and rebellion, and that women were partaking in such an existence in equal numbers to the men.

The Spice Girls with their impossible-to-ignore proclamation of 'Girl Power', saw their debut hit, 'Wannabe', shoot to number one in 1996 in more than thirty countries, propelling the band to superstardom. Their debut album, *Spice*, went on to become the biggest-selling album by a female group in history with thirty million copies being sold worldwide. Their fame and colossal success was due in no small way to the notion of female empowerment the band promoted which held great appeal to young girls, teenagers and grown women alike. The Spice Girls were the mainstream manifestation of the undercurrent of the ladette culture – these five feisty young women, Sporty, Baby, Posh, Scary, and Ginger, articulated the trend of sexy, bolshie, empowered females to the whole world.

Shortly after the explosion that was the Spice Girls, I entered into a relationship with the man who was to become my husband. We started 'dating', although back then in the world I inhabited the origins of romance were less to do with actively going on any dates and more to do with getting drunk with a large crowd, before snogging, inebriated and oblivious to those nearby, in a dark corner of the pub. After six months of being a couple I discovered I was pregnant. It was 1998, and I proceeded to drop out of university, get a job as a nursing assistant and move in with my betrothed.

My experience of pregnancy and the resultant motherhood was one of a sharp distinction between the expectations and assumptions of a ladette, caught up in the zeitgeist of Girl Power as extolled by the Spice Girls, and a resounding return to real life, prompted by the cries of a new-born baby, distressingly vibrant stretch marks, and piles of dirty laundry.

Here's the thing: women born in the 1970s were raised to feel like equals. We took this parity for granted as it was our mothers who had first tasted the bittersweet balancing act of childcare, housework, and employment, something which we therefore grew up entirely accustomed to. Popular culture had played its part during our childhoods in reinforcing the ideology that women are fully capable of living life to the full, of maxing out on recreation and fun instead of worrying about our reputations or finding Mr Right, as our grandmothers might have done.

As I sang alongside my group of male and female friends to 'Football's Coming Home' by the Three Lions during one of the matches of Euro '96, drunk on Stella Artois and high on life, I was equal in every way to the male members of the group. With no children between us and a hippy-like, egalitarian view of the world, there was nothing which could have tipped the balance of equality; alcohol, football, good times, no responsibilities – common threads that bound us together for a brief period before the traditional roles of husband, wife, mum, and dad would begin to creep up on us, insidiously removing all that we assumed was ours for the keeping.

My husband wasn't sexist, I should state at this juncture. He emanated from the same social scenes that I had, with identical cultural influences, ideologies and dreams for the future which were pretty much in line with my own. However, with the raw and primal nature of childbirth comes a startling return to more traditional roles for many couples, and we were no exception to the rule.

If we argued, he was the one who got to storm out and head for the pub and a gallon of lager to sooth away his new fatherhood-related worries and stress. I remained trapped in our flat with a screaming baby who, more often than not, sported a crimson face due to severe episodes of colic. As I had resigned from my job as nursing assistant around the thirty-five weeks pregnant stage, I was not so much on maternity leave but rather an unlimited period of full-time motherhood. He was in the early stages of building a creative design empire and with little money between us derived from just one source of income (his), ninety per cent of the childcare responsibilities naturally fell into my lap.

Looking back on the first few weeks of Isobel's life, I think I was relieved to a degree that the constant drinking and partying had taken a back seat, and I felt content and happy to be a mother. There were difficult moments and I had nowhere near the emotional reserves to draw upon I do today (as mum for the second time around, to toddler Lily), but for the majority of the time I settled contentedly into a very traditional role. Maybe hormones played their part but I don't remember feeling restless or suffering pangs of rebellion against my new life in the early days – other than when my husband and I had a fight and he would leave me to deal with the weighty responsibilities of parenthood alone, and then the unfairness of the situation would rise up like a wild storm and knock me sideways.

We fell into a whole new world of nappies, breastfeeding, prams, walks in the park, having a much-reduced social life, shopping trips to Mothercare and family holidays to Center Parcs, and as my husband beavered away in the corner of the living room building his business, I established friendships with a group of women who had all had babies at around the same time as me.

As the weeks turned into months, things gradually began to return to how they'd been pre-pregnancy, albeit in a slightly curtailed, modified fashion to accommodate the fact that we were now three rather than two. We began to socialise once again, sometimes together when we had managed to find a willing babysitter, and on other occasions we would go out alone with our respective friends. This gave rise to a male/female divide which had remained absent throughout the last few years of my life but which, with parenthood, was beginning to emerge as standard. The weekends became about 'girls' nights out' and 'lads' nights out'; for me, these weekly respites from domesticity meant getting dolled up, drunk, and very loud.

We were now in the last year of the millennium, and social nuances had shifted a gear since the mid-1990s when the pint-swigging ladette was having her heyday. In 1996 Helen Fielding's *Bridget Jones's Diary* was published, later to be made into a film in 2001. The effect that the Bridget Jones phenomenon had upon the drinking habits of women belonging to a certain demographic should not be underplayed, and I was most definitely whipped along in this chardonnay tailspin as I resumed my social life as a new mother.

Bridget's diary was full to the brim of her failed efforts to stick to healthy eating and drinking patterns. Her calorie content far exceeded her dieter's limitations and all attempts to avoid (or at least keep to a minimum) alcohol and cigarettes largely went out of the window as she tried valiantly to cope with the stresses of life as a female singleton in London.

It was this notion of trying but failing that most struck a chord with the women who lapped up Fielding's literary creation in their droves; Jones represented the human failings in all of us, it wasn't that she didn't know about the harms of alcohol or cigarettes, or that she wasn't aware of the fact that she was a few pounds overweight, but it was the fact that her New Year's resolutions proved so difficult to stick to that caused us to love her so much. The postfeminist single women of the Western world were delighted to discover a modern-day heroine who was so honest and comical in her struggles to keep within government alcohol guidelines, her two-fingers-up-to-the-world attitude which manifested itself in the greedy swigs she took from a vodka bottle, and the way in which nights out with her urban friends automatically involved drinking to reach a state of oblivion.

Sick of being patronised and told how to behave by the perceived 'Nanny State', grown-up women were suddenly given *carte blanche* to rebel a little – alcohol, and in particular white wine (Bridget Jones's favourite tipple was chardonnay) was portrayed as an easy and effective tool for achieving this aim. Bridget was an intelligent, educated, and independent woman who was not afraid of doing as she pleased. This was not a down-and-out, drinking cider on a park bench, but a journalist who drew the gaze of attractive men such as Mark Darcy and Daniel Cleaver (played by Colin Firth and Hugh Grant respectively); a woman who had funny and cool friends, a woman with attitude, a woman with wine.

At the same time, HBO's *Sex and the City* was gathering momentum as a similarly postfeminist take on metropolitan life for thirty-something women. Broadcast between 1998 and 2004, viewers were presented with author Candace Bushnell's protagonists; Carrie Bradshaw, Samantha Jones, Charlotte York and Miranda Hobbes – respectively, a fashion-obsessed newspaper columnist, a sexually-confident PR-based businesswoman, a woman of a privileged background who worked in an art gallery, and a feminist, somewhat cynical, lawyer. When socialising together, these four women were routinely depicted in achingly cool bars and restaurants around downtown

Manhattan as they shared intimate details of their exciting adventures in love with one another over fancy cocktails.

The women whom I was friends with around this time were virtually all grown-up ladettes, veterans of the rave scene who were now married with babies. Set against the cultural landscape of *Sex and the City* and *Bridget Jones's Diary*, we enthusiastically cemented our friendships in fashionable bars and clubs at the weekends, where we drank colossal amounts before stumbling home in the small hours, trying not to wake our sleeping children and husbands. We holidayed together, and spent Sunday afternoons in pub beer gardens with our families. Here we never grew too drunk as our children were present but still, alcohol always featured heavily on the agenda.

Gradually my tastes altered during the first couple of years of Isobel's life, from pints of lager to exclusively white wine. I was happy to be a mum, but the alcohol I drank provided me with a means of hanging on to the old me. And opting for wine allowed me to remain entirely free of feelings of guilt over the regularity and volume of alcohol that I was consuming.

Wine, though, was not a beverage that I grew up believing to be a staple of daily life. With Sunday dinner my parents took pleasure in a single bottle of German wine, Liebfraumilch usually, and my sister and I were granted a tiny sip each, 'just a taste'. As a family we would visit friends in Frankfurt, Germany, from time to time and the manner in which wine formed a more integral part of life there perhaps rubbed off on my mum and dad a little. The notion that occasionally allowing children a thimbleful of wine would assist them in older years to approach alcohol responsibly was at the forefront of my parents' thinking when pouring us a small amount, an idea they more than likely picked up when holidaying on the Continent.

However, my parents' kitchen was never home to

multiple bottles of wine, stacked up neatly on display in a stylish wine rack. Wine was not something which was brought out on a whim, mid-week to be slugged down thirstily only to be swiftly followed by the popping of a second cork. And yet as a mother and young woman in my mid-twenties, wine had become an absolutely vital element of my own family's weekly grocery shop – I thought nothing of the health implications of all that booze and far more about which flavour would best suit each meal, of whether my knowledge of wines was ample enough to demonstrate the certain sophistication that I was seeking. The fact that our alcohol budget ran into the hundreds each month did nothing to deter my husband and me from drinking so readily.

Wine did not register in my conscience as a dangerous, toxic, or unhealthy liquid. Consuming it helped me to feel grown-up and normal, and I never for a moment considered doing otherwise. With hindsight I recognise how alcohol had become the key ingredient in preventing any onset of 'frumpiness' or boredom from setting in. My life had become the usual treadmill of domestic chores; making the beds, washing the clothes, preparing dinner, shopping, changing nappies, bathing the baby, vacuuming and tidying, and yet with the promise of wine never far from my mind I plodded on through the daylight hours while reassuring myself that as soon as all the necessary housework and mothering was behind me, the 'me time' could commence.

Mid-week drinking was a precursor to the weekend blowouts, enough to satisfy any yearnings for mild escapism but not sufficient to seriously impact on my ability to get up in the mornings, back in the role of Mum. And it would appear that I was not alone in my domiciliary drinking habits.

A 2009 Joseph Rowntree Foundation review of research relevant to trends in alcohol consumption over a twenty to thirty year period highlighted a marked increase in the overall level of binge-drinking in women. The report showed that the number of women who engaged in binge-drinking almost doubled from eight per cent in 1998 to fifteen per cent in 2006, with a more pronounced increase in those over the age of twenty-five. This was compared to an overall reduction in the number of UK men binge-drinking during the same period. Patterns in the behaviour of young people also showed a decrease in the numbers binge-drinking. So, as the rest of society either remained the same as recent years in terms of volume and regularity of binge-drinking or evidenced a decline, women dramatically upped their booze game.

Alcohol almost certainly played a part in helping me to gloss over various traumas I'd experienced as I matured into adulthood; a dogged eating disorder (almost fully resolved with the discovery that I was expecting a baby, and the resultant wish to nurture my unborn daughter) and becoming entangled in a violent relationship with an older man who bullied and abused me. My female friends had all been through the mill somewhat too, with miscarriages, abortions, rape, and post-natal depression to throw into the amalgamation of our collective history.

Abiding by an unspoken convention of 'putting up and shutting up' neither my friends nor I openly aired any grievances over the difficulties we had lived through. We nodded to the fact that such incidences had taken place, usually when drunk and sharing yet another bottle of wine, smoking heavily and leaning into one another in the dark corner of a bar. But we were somehow resigned to the fact that this was life, the bad stuff occurred no matter who you were or where you came from, and none of it credited you with the right to let it drag you down.

The preferred coping strategy was wine, and large amounts thereof. We drank to blot out the pain of the past, and we drank to enable ourselves to live up to who we thought we should be. We drank to cling on to the young girl with bags of freedom, who had so miraculously been replaced by an adult woman bothered by such demands as planning a week's worth of healthy meals for the family, keeping the bathroom clean, and providing endless entertainment for energetic toddlers.

In an ideal world I would have dealt with my various 'issues' as they'd occurred but instead I buried them beneath a hectic social life. Years later when I undertook a course of therapy sessions, the counsellor informed me that my emotions appeared to have been frozen at about the age of fifteen. This was when my life began to revolve around using drugs and alcohol to the point of total obliteration on most weekends. It was when I had ceased to consciously process my feelings – deaths, relationship break-ups, my eating disorder and other challenges had been tipped into a compartment of my mind and left to fester for many years.

Unwittingly, wine became my medicine and without it I would no doubt have been more aware of the responsibilities of motherhood that now faced me. As a drinker, I lacked any acceptance of how life had changed, and how having a baby and being married *should* quite rightly have altered me and my behaviour. So accustomed was I to living the high life and shirking all cares of what the future may hold, I did not conceive for a single moment that it was time for all the wildness and the parties to come to an end. It was merely a case of adjusting, fine-tuning, and tweaking to ensure that, baby notwithstanding, life carried on pretty much as it always had.

Ann Dowsett Johnston claims that "We live in an alcogenic culture, one where risky drinking has been normalized. We swim in an ocean of advertising, and that advertising says one thing: drink, and great things will happen. We absorb this in our pores. In fact, it's so prevalent, we barely notice it."[8] Western society does indeed endorse binge-drinking, and following on from the cultural female icons of the Spice Girls, Bridget Jones, and Carrie Bradshaw et al in *Sex and the City*, women during the noughties were comfortable acting with bravado and balls in a way their mothers had not.

The ladette phenomenon coupled with more aggressively female-targeted advertising by the alcohol industry (especially with regards to spirits and wine) during the 1990s led to an easy and relaxed regard for hazardous drinking patterns. The overriding sense that drinking such vast amounts of booze was perfectly normal meant that personally I did not question the level of my consumption, and failed to take on board just how much of a negative impact alcohol was having – both on my ability to be a parent, and on my personality and approach to life.

Growing up surrounded by the victories of the second-wave feminist movement, with a mother who, along with almost all her peers had a career *and* simultaneously raised a family *and* took care of all the household chores, and went about it all with such aplomb that I never stopped for a second to consider what damn hard work it all amounted to, I failed to accurately foresee that challenges that lay ahead of me as a parent. I expected wholeheartedly and with absolutely no consideration of the alternative that I would be happy and fulfilled as a mother and wife, and that I would have a husband who'd stick by me and support my dreams with love and devotion, just as my dad had always done for my mum.

I'd lived a free and irresponsible existence for as long as I had been independent. Reckless, impetuous and hedonistic, by the time I was married at the young age of twenty-three, my perception of life was firmly focused on fun and entertainment. I imagine my grandmothers and

---

[8] [8] Drink, The Intimate Relationship Between Women and Alcohol, Ann Dowsett Johnston, Fourth Estate, 2013, p. 233.

even my mother would have possessed utterly different notions of what married life involved on the eve of their wedding days; for me, it was all about excitement, romance, booze, parties, and continuing the glory days for ever. And because alcohol had featured so strongly in the years preceding our marriage, it was this magical substance that I looked to for the provision of all the good times that I was sure lay ahead.

As a person who regularly drank alcohol I was driven to turn each and every occasion into a booze-fuelled blast – this was all as a result of subconscious mental meanderings and never a desire which I recognised until I quit drinking for good. But I was unable to just *be*, to enjoy a quiet evening alone with a book, or to spend the weekend walking in the countryside (minus the pub at the end of the walk in which several pints of ale would more than likely be downed). I was running from something, perpetually keeping my demons at bay, and therefore unable to accept the life of a housewife and mother as my lot.

Older generations had faced the same challenges, boredom, and frustrations as my own but they had been without the taste of true equality that had seemed so real to me, pre-parenthood. Not only had both my grandmothers lived very different, less hedonistic lifestyles as teenagers and young women, but the second-wave feminist movement had yet to embed itself in the social climate when they were starting out as married women. Women had none of the purchasing power or economic freedom that is more characteristic of their younger counterparts. A college education was not accepted as the norm in the way it is today; in fact one of my grandmothers left school at the age of fourteen, working for a few years on a local farm before marrying at the age of twenty-one.

Expectations were vastly different from those of modern-day women and although I thought I was coasting along nicely during Isobel's infancy and early childhood, with hindsight it was largely because most nights I was numbing any underlying boredom and lack of self-fulfilment with booze.

The change in the drinking behaviours of Western women born in the latter half of the twentieth century is evidenced in research conducted by the University of Washington. The study pinpointed women who were born after World War II as experiencing more alcohol dependence than earlier generations. Led by Richard A. Grucza, the researchers examined the 1991 and 1992 National Longitudinal Alcohol Epidemiologic Survey (NLAES), and the National Epidemiological Survey on Alcohol and Related Conditions (NESARC), conducted in 2001 and 2002.

"We found that for women born after World War II, there are lower levels of abstaining from alcohol, and higher levels of alcohol dependence, even when looking only at women who drank," said Grucza. "However, we didn't see any significant tendency for more recently born men to have lower levels of abstention, or higher levels of alcohol dependence." The results suggest a closing of the gender gap in alcohol dependency.

It would seem that as the female population has enjoyed an increase in economic and social equality alongside a broadening of opportunities which simply didn't exist for women born in earlier years, so too we have come to perceive alcohol as an integral element of our advanced freedoms. The growth in recent decades of sales of wine and vodka, both beverages traditionally more popular with women, further evidences this trend. In addition, the explosion of alcoholic drinks specifically engineered to appeal to the female market illustrates what the booze industry knows all too well; women are more often than not the ones with the household purchasing power.

Feminism has delivered many things for women during recent times but one thing it has not granted us is immunity to the harms of heavy and regular binge-drinking. Low to moderate alcohol consumption has been linked to a statistical increase in cancer risks, notably cancers of the breast, liver, rectum, and upper aero-digestive tract combined. The Million Women Study is a national (UK) study of women's health involving more than 1,000,000 women aged fifty plus. Cancer Research UK and the National Health Service are joint collaborators on the project, which is being run by Oxford University. The Million Women Study has found that in developed countries like the UK, the lifetime risk of having breast cancer is 1 in 8. For every extra daily alcoholic drink consumed, that risk increases by 1.1 per 100. So if you had a roughly 12.5% chance of getting breast cancer, but you drank one glass of wine a day, that risk would go up to 13.6%. If you drank two glasses of wine a day, that would increase to 14.7%.

These might sound like quite small increases in risk. But because many women drink alcohol at these sorts of levels, it means a lot of women are affected overall. It is estimated that alcohol accounts for 11% of all breast cancers in the UK. That means that every year, 5,000 women get breast cancer who wouldn't have got it without drinking alcohol. And breast cancer is on the rise; it is the most common cancer in the UK and the incidence rate has been steadily moving upwards for several years.

In 1999, 42,400 women were diagnosed with the disease. Almost a decade later in 2008, 47,700 women were found to have breast cancer. With the changing size of the population being accounted for, this is an increase of around 3.5 per cent in the breast cancer incidence rate.[9]

[9] Statistics from Cancer Research UK –
http://scienceblog.cancerresearchuk.org/2011/02/04/why-are-breast-cancer-rates-increasing/.

There *are* serious physical repercussions to drinking heavily as a woman and these are increasingly coming to light. In the years between 2002 and 2012 the number of women in the UK admitted to hospital due to alcohol-related incidents doubled nationwide. The female body is not able to process alcohol as effectively as the male, and with smaller frames meaning less tissue to absorb alcohol plus a higher ratio of fat to water women are less able to dilute alcohol within the body, so the consequences of alcohol are more severe.

Alcohol-related liver disease is the major cause of overall liver disease in the Western world. Of those who develop it (in England in 2011/12 there were 49,456 hospital admissions for alcohol-related liver disease[10]) women are twice as susceptible as men and may develop the disease as a result of a shorter duration and dose of chronic alcohol consumption. This gender difference could be explained by less alcohol dehydrogenase in the gut, a higher proportion of body fat as well as changes in fat absorption due to the menstrual cycle.

As previously stated, women are not physiologically equal to men when it comes to alcohol consumption. As intelligent and educated individuals most of us are mindful of this fact, and yet there is something about the bottle which keeps drawing us back time and time again. I was not in the dark about alcohol being an addictive substance, I knew that it can cause depression, and I had begun in the years immediately preceding my last drink to develop an awareness regarding the connection between breast cancer and booze. On occasion, the fear that I might have brought about untold numbers of diseases and afflictions as a result of my lifestyle choices would grip me, my mind running away with awful imaginings of premature and painful

[10] Statistic from the Alcohol Concern UK – http://www.alcoholconcern.org.uk/campaign/statistics-on-alcohol

death scenarios.

But I didn't stop drinking.

Societies of developed countries are heavily weighted towards drinking alcohol; it is cheap, freely available, and routinely presented as a totally acceptable way to relax and have fun, adding a little glamour and pizzazz to events or a night out with the girls. It is also seriously addictive. The ubiquitous nature of booze made it virtually impossible for me to conceive that this magic potion, which had been a part of every aspect of my life since my teens, could *really* be doing me some damage. The people who suffered the ill consequences of alcohol were surely those in parks drinking from supersize bottles of cider, the *alcoholics*, anyone but me. The denial was all-consuming; so long as I continued to absorb the positive messages about alcohol as presented by the world at large, and maintained a mental division of the ones who were in trouble with booze and people like me, I was protected from the harms of drinking.

Throughout the last twenty years women have been sold a myth; that wine is a treat, a source of respite from the daily domestic grind, a rope that links us to our halcyon youth amidst the turbulent waters of middle-age. We have been conditioned to believe that as we pour a glass of chilled white or room-temperature red we are securing our social status as sophisticated, knowledgeable, middle-class grown-ups. We possess the wine education necessary for recognising that a light, quaffable merlot pairs nicely with pasta dishes and roast chicken, but that a fuller bodied, riper style can complement beautifully a spicy meal such as jambalaya. Nights with the girls would be unthinkable without an ample stock of white, red, or rose, the following morning's hangover as much of a thing to share a laugh over as the evening's drunken shenanigans themselves. The idea that alcohol can wrap a blanket of comfort and tranquillity around us at the end of a manic day juggling a career, children, and housework is one that millions have bought into.

But with over three years of living without alcohol behind me, I know that the above are nothing but persuasive yet false ideals, drilled into our consciousness so effectively and insidiously that we, more often than not, fail to even notice how much of our minds and bodies we have sacrificed in the name of booze.

As a mother I was regularly bad-tempered and snappy as a direct consequence of drinking too much alcohol. This is not as harmless an effect as it may sound but a trend which, over the course of my older daughter's childhood prevented the two of us from being as close as we might otherwise have been. Bedtime stories being delivered without the reader (i.e. me) rushing along in order to break away in haste for a glass of wine, moments of uncertainty or reservation which should have been resolved with a cuddle from Mummy, pleas to stay up for just ten more minutes at bedtime as a rare treat – these things should be absolutely guaranteed for any little girl but were too often forsaken in the name of white wine. A request to go swimming, or to take the ball down to the park for an energetic kick about, or a desire to dig out the arts and crafts box, make an almighty and gluey mess and enjoy being creative together; simple activities that bond parent and child but which don't happen when Mummy has a crippling hangover and can barely manage to shift from the settee.

The glass, or more usually, the bottle of wine did not manifest any true degree of relaxation or a recharging of the batteries as promised when I utilized it as a frazzled mother. The alcohol affected me in a number of ways, but predominantly it was the depressive episodes and anxiety attacks, the lethargy caused by hangovers, and the lack of tolerance which wielded the most disruption and damage in my relationship with Isobel.

I also believe that the almost daily popping of the cork at 7 p.m. signalled a definite ending of the period of full accessibility to Mum – the wine demarcated the close of the daily grind and the beginning of 'adult time'. I became a different person when I drank alcohol and am certain that this shift in my personality would not have gone unnoticed by Isobel as a small child, even if she was too young to fully acknowledge what was going on.

Last week, two-year-old Lily needed an activity to prevent her from climbing the walls, beset as we had been by torrential downpours. I filled the kitchen sink with bubbly water, wrapped an over-size apron around her and added a few plastic containers and spoons to the washing-up bowl for her to play with. As she perched on the chair, leaning forwards and pouring away to her heart's content, I stood next to her and was completely drawn into her magnificent little world. Her blue eyes revealed mammoth levels of concentration as she busily swapped one container for another, tipped some water down the waste-disposal section, stirred a little here and there, poured some more. For an hour I stood by her side next to the sink, observing her, filled with love and affection, allowing her to explore and grow and feel excitement at the ordinary and the everyday.

I would not have acted in this way back in my drinking days. I'd have been hungover, grumpy, tired, and ultimately resentful of having to keep my child entertained when really what I craved was a few hours in bed followed by a restful afternoon with a magazine and several cups of tea. The wine I'd have knocked back the night before would have resulted in me not sharing this moment of closeness with Lily. If I'd bothered at all to go to the trouble of setting her up with some washing-up fun I'd have barked when she'd accidentally spilled some water, tutted at her for soaking her clothes, and huffed and puffed as I'd cleaned up the spillage afterwards. Drawn out over an entire childhood, these characteristics have an impact.

A further improvement to my parenting abilities as a consequence of quitting drinking is that I have finally, and with a great deal of effort, put to rest my various longstanding 'issues'. Because I no longer smother all my emotions with booze I am a less angry, bitter person who has more headspace to think of others and a greater capacity for empathy. I have drawn a line in the sand with regards to my divorce. The pain and loneliness that I endured for years as a single parent have vanished and the experience of living through that period has provided me with a degree of humility, gratitude for things I may otherwise have taken for granted, and a desire to not make the same mistakes with my current relationship as I did in my marriage.

I have also grasped the concept that it is possible to be a woman and not be a victim. The ups and downs of life as an alcohol-dependent singleton who was attempting to blunt the sharp edges with booze, men, and partying, no longer appeal to me. I have no wish to seek pleasure or satisfaction outside of the things in my life that are of the utmost importance. Being a good mum, fulfilling my potential, sustaining a happy and equal relationship with my partner Sean, and trying to be a good person who thinks of others are the things that make me happy and the most content.

I am now a strong and mentally together person who looks after her family and who values motherhood as a vital role which makes a world of difference when done properly. I accept that my days are often filled with a certain element of chaos as I spin the many plates of managing Soberistas, writing, childcare, housework, relationships, wider family, seeing friends, running, and so on. But the perception that all of this equates to me somehow being put upon, of unfairness and relentless demands being thrust on me that I cannot cope with has disappeared. This is my lot, I'm a woman and I choose to have this life – I wanted my children and I also enjoy working, and without alcohol skewing the balance none of it is that hard to manage any more.

A practical benefit of not drinking is that I now have approximately thirty hours of additional time in which to work, organise things like meal-planning, do the supermarket shop, go running, enjoy a night of quality time with my older daughter, or do anything else I fancy. Instead of permanently feeling as though I am up against it, that life is a race against time and that attending to such annoyances as sorting through unwanted clothes or taking old toys to the charity shop is something that merely gets in the way of drinking, life has taken on a more manageable feel. I remain on top of stuff, mostly, and this is reflected in healthier and more budget-friendly family meals, a tidier house, and ultimately, an increase in the time I can spend on things like helping Isobel with her homework, playing with Lily, or taking the dog for a good long walk.

One final point to make on the subject of women and alcohol: we are prone to particular secondary harms of drinking that either do not affect men, or do so but not to the same degree. This includes contracting STDs, as a woman's anatomy can increase the risk factor for STD infection compared to men because the lining of the vagina is thinner and more delicate than the skin on the penis thus enabling bacteria and viruses to penetrate more easily. In addition, the moistness of the vaginal area provides a good environment for the growth of bacteria.[11] There is also the risk of being the victims of sexual abuse and domestic violence, and experiencing unwanted pregnancies. Alcohol, when consumed excessively, damages both our fertility and our unborn babies (Foetal Alcohol Syndrome

---

[11] See http://www.cdc.gov/nchhstp/newsroom/docs/STDs-Women-042011.pdf

and an increased risk of miscarriage), and it also exaggerates some menopausal side-effects.

As a teenager and young woman, being a feminist was all about keeping up with the boys in the pub and living the high life with no real thought for anyone but me. As someone who is now on the brink of turning forty I am very proud of my womanhood, of being a good mum, of my exceptional daughters, and of my passion for life without alcohol.

I am not a victim; I am a strong and capable woman.

Chapter Six – Love Thyself

"The most terrifying thing is to accept oneself completely."
– C.G. Jung

Sex for me had, almost without exception, taken place through a blurry alcohol-fuelled lens ever since I became sexually active in my mid-teens. Sex with my now-ex-husband was no different, but with the added strains and pressures that go hand-in-hand with parenthood there were multiple reasons why booze seemed all the more essential in any bedroom antics we engaged in. Firstly, I had developed bright red, angry-looking stretch marks all across my stomach and thighs during the latter weeks of my pregnancy. Secondly, the ensuing protracted labour had culminated in an epidural, forceps, and an episiotomy which was so painful I'd had to breastfeed lying down in bed for the first six weeks of Isobel's life owing to being unable to sit upright in a chair. Both of these factors led to a serious reduction in body confidence.

Thirdly (and connected to the first two issues) I went off the idea of sex for quite some time. In my mind, intimate coupling inevitably concluded with the agonising and exhausting event that is childbirth – the concept that the act of sex might occur purely on the basis that one was turned on and it felt good had been disposed of along with the last remnants of the placenta.

How then, did I overcome these barriers to getting down to business beneath the duvet as a young mum, aged twenty-three? Simple – alcohol.

Back then I don't think I was particularly, if at all aware of the fact that alcohol served as a fast-track ticket to physical togetherness. It was such an integral and natural part of my world that the various feelings it usually induced such as loosening me up, reducing my inhibitions, or sparking a degree of sexiness (at least before the tipping point was reached and it all raced away down a steep hill of puking, stumbling, and falling unconscious) did not register with me. But I subconsciously relied upon booze as a method of igniting that desire, and if it had not been a part of the equation then our sex life as a young married couple would most probably have been non-existent – at least for those early years of Isobel's life. From romantic weekends away (minus baby) to special meals cooked at home, all our efforts to keep alive the flame of attraction amidst the humdrum of domestic life were awash with booze.

There were several factors behind my limited body confidence following the birth of my first child, and all had been bubbling away under the surface for quite some years. I hadn't been especially troubled by shyness in the bedroom or a lack of desire previously because alcohol had always been there as a magic solution to buoy up my sexual prowess. However, with a newborn baby sharing our bedroom and an alcohol-free existence due to breastfeeding I was suddenly conscious of not being 'in the mood', and of all my perceived physical shortcomings.

As young girls we often experience a creeping sense of not being good or pretty enough, which throughout our teenage years gradually chips away at the belief we held as children that we're actually OK. As a child I gave little heed to my appearance (although I did have a penchant for wearing several different outfits throughout the course of the day, much to my mother's dismay when wash day came around!) and was not particularly plagued by any notions of being ugly, fat, or somehow below par

128

physically.

And then in my early teens I took on board the idea that I was fat or at least that if I wasn't careful of my diet then I would certainly become that way. I began to avoid meals, weighing myself several times a day and making myself sick whenever I 'gave in' and ate something. My weight plummeted and by the age of sixteen the scales were hovering around the six and a half stone mark. I was disgusted by my own body and would grab at my flesh in front of the mirror, repelled by what was, by then, just skin and essential tissue. I was overly sensitive to any remarks that were remotely related to fatness and greed even if they were not aimed my way. My mood was shot to pieces, a combination of teenage hormones, alcohol and drug use, and my strict 'diet' resulting in malnutrition and the occasional fainting episode. It all contributed to a fractured mental state.

My eating disorder was to stay with me to varying degrees for the next seven years and was something I only managed to conquer with the discovery that I was pregnant with Isobel. The commonly heard advice of not drinking alcohol on an empty stomach was somewhat irrelevant to me in my mid to late teens; virtually the only calories I took on came in liquid form and I'd developed a reasonably high tolerance of booze which meant I could usually hold my drink despite not having eaten anything for days at a time.

I knew a few girls around that time who were similarly affected by eating disorders and who drank excessively. For me, and I suspect for them too, food wasn't an option because it was solid, thus appearing more likely to cause weight gain, but beer and wine came with the pretence of containing no calories and were apparently therefore 'allowed'. Alcohol also fired up low self-confidence and provided a respite from the obsessive and never-ending internal ruminations about food, weight, diets, and the fear of growing obese. Getting drunk brought about a little holiday from the tortuous mental gymnastics of my mind.

Scrutinizing one's physical form consistently with a fear of fatness colouring everyday life is a difficult habit to break. In addition the fact that I had, pre-pregnancy, attempted to remedy such pervasive and negative thought patterns with booze heightened the association I had of alcohol as a mood-enhancer. Low body confidence and drinking were inextricably linked, to the extent that during pregnancy and the first weeks of Isobel's life when booze was off the menu I found the act of looking at myself naked excruciating – the visible signs of pregnancy coupled with the lack of ethanol by which to numb how I was feeling led to vastly increased unhappiness with my body (or at least, that's how it felt; not much had changed in reality in that I'd never been satisfied with my appearance but previously booze had done a reasonably decent job of masking those thoughts).

I despised my legs, in particular my thighs, and refused to wear skirts or dresses that sat above the knee. I avoided mirrors when naked, and bathing was an activity that led to serious levels of self-hatred with regards to my body. I wasn't comfortable with intimacy, and a significant element of this was because I had no idea how to behave minus the disinhibiting effects of alcohol. I felt depressed and unhappy with my shape, and could find no part of it which I was content with. I felt obligated to eat well and regularly as I was breastfeeding, but never fully stopped wishing I was thinner.

And all of this was occurring when I was just eleven and a half stone at nine months pregnant, and back down to a healthy ten stone a couple of months after giving birth.

Not everyone goes through an eating disorder, but countless women in the West are similarly critical of their appearance to a degree, so much so that in December 2012 equalities minister Jo Swinson felt compelled to write an open letter to the editors of various UK publications asking that they drop the features on 'miracle diets' and adopt an overall more responsible approach to how women's bodies are represented within magazines.

In an interview with the *Guardian* newspaper about her campaign, Swinson said, "The imagery that we're presented with has just one type of so-called ideal which is very, very slim, generally very, very young as well, late teens or early 20s, and it is something which is unattainable and, indeed, not reflective of the true diversity of beauty that's out there.

"So when your sister or your friend is standing there and moaning about whether she looks really fat, and actually she looks gorgeous, tell her so and support each other. Very often this kind of criticism, and self-criticism, is something which goes unchallenged and I think there's a resolution there for everyone to challenge that default setting."[12]

The emphasis on thinness as an essential ingredient of beauty (as purported by the media at large) is a relatively recent phenomenon; it wasn't until the 1990s that the excessive promotion of waif-like bodies began to be established as the norm. Twiggy arrived on the 1960s fashion scene with a Body Mass Index (BMI) of just 14.7, signalling the beginning of a trend towards thinner models, but mid-twentieth century curvy women continued to be celebrated for their attractiveness for decades to come. Marilyn Monroe's much revered hourglass figure (BMI of around 20) represented a female form which was far from emaciated, and she has maintained her status as sex goddess into the twenty-first century.

A shift in the female body shape considered most

---

[12] See http://www.guardian.co.uk/lifeandstyle/2012/dec/27/women-weight-minister-jo-swinson

fashionable is illustrated in the Miss America beauty pageant records. During the 1920s, the average waist measurement was 25.3 (between the years of 1921 and 1927). In the 1980s the average was 23.3 and three of the 1980s contestants' waists measured a minuscule 22 inches. On the catwalk, Kate Moss sparked headlines in the 1990s for her skeletal appearance, and later Lily Cole, Victoria Beckham, and Nicole Ritchie were all poster girls for the 'size zero' body which led to outcries for fashion houses to employ only models with figures that reflected those in the real world.[13]

During the latter part of the twentieth century, Western women were influenced by an obsession with a female form which is young, child-like, and thin. A number of those who have been instrumental in promoting a more realistic body shape (for instance Sophie Dahl) have witnessed success and a high public profile, but the media persists in promoting super slim women as normal, often with facial and bodily characteristics which are wholly unattainable due to the fact that they are either fake or computer-enhanced (adverts from cosmetics company L'Oreal were banned in 2011 as they were found to feature airbrushed images of actress Julia Roberts and model Christy Turlington).

With such a persistent refusal amongst those in the media to acknowledge the diverse nature of the real life female body, and a prescriptive ideal of what it allegedly takes for us to be considered beautiful, it comes as no great shock that many women feel unhappy with their physicality. Alcohol serves many of us in our quest to inject some body confidence as well as helping to reduce our sexual inhibitions, making us feel seductive and more

---

[13] See http://www.pbs.org/wgbh/amex/missamerica/sfeature/sf_l ist.html

daring in intimate situations.

As we mature into adults we are educated on matters of the bedroom via popular culture. On films and the television we are supplied with the recipe for sexual success, and it is repeated and reflected across the entire cultural spectrum. We see slim, glamorous females in slinky lingerie sipping alcoholic drinks and behaving in a tantalizing fashion (remember *Pretty Woman* in which Julia Roberts gets giggly and alluring on champagne before working her sexual magic on a non-drinking Richard Gere?) We are privy to untold numbers of female film leads drinking to the point of oblivion before rolling into bed with their male counterpart (Cameron Diaz springs to mind in her role in *The Holiday* – drinking until unconscious we then find her struggling to piece together the previous night's activities with Jude Law, something he clearly finds enchanting and cute).

In *Friends,* Rachel and Ross get blind drunk in Las Vegas and tie the knot, an event which neither one remembers fully in the morning and which we, as the audience, are intended to find hilarious. James Bond, the archetypal smooth-talking womaniser, is rarely seen in a romantic situation without his beloved martini, 'shaken, not stirred'. And the king of the 1980s pin ups, Tom Cruise, delivered his impassioned 'The Last Barman Poet' to an enraptured audience in the 1988 movie *Cocktail,* while simultaneously making 'fuck-me eyes' (his words, not mine) at the woman of his dreams who is watching him with awe.

Sex is powerful stuff and we live in a society saturated with alcohol-related sexual imagery and messages. Women in films are frequently portrayed as letting their hair down, dancing erotically, and acting with sexual bravado following a few drinks; we commonly see men acting in a sophisticated, James Bond-esque manner, authoritative and masculine in their approach to pursuing a love interest.

By the time we reach eighteen it is hardly surprising that boozing and bonking appear to go hand in hand. I certainly never questioned this connection and dutifully set about purchasing bottles of wine whenever I invited a boyfriend around for a romantic evening. When drinking alcohol, the boost to low sexual confidence is palpable – it can be felt coursing around one's body almost instantaneously after sipping from that first glass. As a result, knowledge of how to act in a sexually confident manner minus the artificial crutch of alcohol is often never learnt, and over time we become increasingly reliant upon alcohol in order to reach that desired state of mind.

In a partnership which is built on the shaky foundations of booze, it isn't just the sex which can be twisted into a false version of reality. Mood swings, infidelities, a mutual lack of trust, and low self-esteem are all common manifestations of the impact alcohol has on us as individuals, and consequently has upon our relationships.

Immediately prior to quitting drinking aged thirty-five, I entered into my only 'grown-up' relationship subsequent to my marriage. For the second time in my adult life I was involved with someone with whom I didn't play mind games, lie to, cheat on, or otherwise piss off monumentally prior to the romance drawing to an unhappy close. Following the end of my marriage my attitude towards men altered dramatically; it is likely that having my fingers burnt in the way I did, when my ex-husband packed his bags and marched off without so much as a word of warning, affected my ability to trust.

But the repeated 'bad relationships' I was involved in between the ages of twenty-eight and thirty-five stemmed from something much deeper than my inherent lack of faith in their longevity, or my trust in men. When I drank alcohol I was selfish, and totally unable to assess my behaviour in a rational fashion. I never did grasp the concept of 'self-sacrifice' prior to becoming a non-drinker and in addition my depressive episodes and terribly low self-esteem conspired to foster a permanent state of discontentment. I always felt as though I was searching for something or someone, even when I had someone – the U2 song 'I Still Haven't Found What I'm Looking For' resonated with me, summarising my restlessness and desire to find it, whatever it may have been.

And when caught up in these romantic unions with all the wrong people I would use alcohol and sex in order to give the relationship meaning and create shared interests, closeness, and a boost to my low confidence. When the early euphoric phase of the relationship had worn off, and niggling doubts would begin to sneak up pertaining to the current Mr Right actually having elements of Mr Wrong about him, I would drink on it. Never go for long walks, have a weekend away by myself to work things out, or even a Saturday night alone at home to enjoy some emotional breathing space; no, when the shit hit the fan out would come the booze, manipulation, tears – and the sexy underwear.

Sex was love back then; it turned the broken and bad into fresh and intact. It was as if the strength of the physical attraction would always serve to wipe out all the things we so obviously did not have in common, together with the numerous issues that made us entirely incompatible. It was a weapon, and in some bizarre combination of narcissism and self-hatred I spent the best part of eight years perceiving myself as reasonably sexually attractive and yet rotten to the core inside. I was unable to believe that by simply being me I could, along with 'normal' people, also be a part of a happy, longstanding relationship. And in being so down on myself and falling into a cycle of short-term flings, I became hooked to the drama of it all – the ups and downs and emotional rollercoaster of not being married, of having the freedoms granted to me every other weekend when Isobel would stay with her dad, of chopping and changing partners whenever I grew tired of them, of repeatedly experiencing the highs of the early stage of relationships.

Despite my addiction to new love interests, there was, ticking along in the recesses of my drink-fuelled, thrill-seeking mind, an unfaltering assumption that Mr Right was out there somewhere – and no matter how impractical or against all odds the union may appear to others I would be right to chase it, to pursue The One when he made his debut on the stage of my life. This perverse idea that Mr Right would not be quite what friends and family were hoping for led me to becoming embroiled in various relationships with unsuitable people: bad boys, a man who lived in a foreign country and with whom I endured several months of a long-distance coupling, and others, details of whom (for the sake of niceties) shall remain undisclosed. I almost actively sought out men who were wrong for me in some way, purely as an act of rebellion.

Alcohol perpetrated this messed-up perception of what it is to be in love. I was, for many years far more in love with the notion of *being* in love than with any of the individuals for whom I professed my uncontrollable desires. The relationships would spark from a boozy initial meeting, and what would more than likely never have been, became something: a togetherness. Drinking allowed me to remain caught up in the fairy tale I was trying so desperately to keep alive – think it, live it, believe it and it will become real.

I drank endless bottles of wine alone in the kitchen during my co-habitation with one boyfriend, and this took place after only a year or two of being with him. Alarm bells failed to ring however and the pinot kept on flowing – nice glass, candle burning, and a glossy magazine to flick through. It never occurred to me that this might not be what true love was all about. In bed, usually slightly tipsy and occasionally hammered on alcohol, everything was just fine.

I was for a long time tangled up in a web of self-made lies and dreamy ideals of what love was all about. Because I had always valued myself so little as a person I placed an unnatural weight of importance on sex, and this had a detrimental effect over the course of my adult life. Caught in a self-fulfilling prophecy, my relationships tended to fare well in the physical stakes, not so well in the emotional or companionship areas. These latter components would be characterised, more often than not, by blazing rows, a deep mistrust of one another, and a lack of shared activities other than those which took place in the pub. Long term this brought me to a frequent conclusion of those with no self-worth; people only wanted me for sex.

Now this wasn't true, but the tragic victim role I tended to lurch towards wanted to believe it, acted upon it, and nurtured the thought until it evolved near enough (at least in my addled mind) into a reality. A common feature of all these relationships in the period between the termination of my marriage and becoming a non-drinker was one of little or no true respect, on either side of the fence; I didn't respect them due to the fact that they 'didn't get me' (not their fault, I just picked the wrong blokes for a while and was usually too pissed or hungover to admit this to either them or myself) and we never had anything in common but getting pissed which led to deep disappointment during the rare times we spent sober. And the various Mr Wrongs did not hold a great deal of respect for me either, certainly as the relationship wore on and my drinking episodes escalated – watching your loved one vomit over the side of the bed, fall over, pass out, and initiate ridiculous and unfounded arguments once too often tends to erode any respect that may have been present in the beginning.

I was driven by a desire to be wanted, in every way,

and when drunk I could almost convince myself that I had obtained what I'd set out to – that my partner was head over heels in love with me. But in the cold light of day the crushing reality of how I regarded myself sober would hit me in waves. If I was ever in attendance of any social situation in which there was a woman younger, prettier, or better dressed than me I would feel desperately jealous, convinced my boyfriend fancied her over me. I felt as though I was nothing, and would drink excessively in order to obliterate the awful feelings of worthlessness.

Under the influence of alcohol I was looser, uninhibited; wearing 'sexy' dressing-up clothes intended to add a certain fruitiness to the occasion, but in which I once became so drunk I toppled off the end of the bed and wound up in a tangle of high heels and bed sheets on the floor, behaving in an unbelievably provocative manner with men who were virtual strangers, throwing myself at them in a way that makes me cringe when I recall it. Various infidelities, engaging in snogging and worse, knowing full well and caring not one jot that I had a trusting partner somewhere back in the real world.

All of these things and more came about because I was devoid of any real sense of self-worth, with a belief that I was sexier when fired-up on drugs or alcohol. I was fortified with the false courage to *act* sexier when high on booze and drugs, and possessed an almost compulsive desire to feel wanted. I do not care to dwell on the number of times that I experienced a complete blackout – a total and utter loss of memory pertaining to several hours of my life. On countless evenings I would be out socialising, drinking heavily, flirting outrageously, on a self-destruct mission and later the next shameful morning have no knowledge of how those inebriated twilight hours had evolved. Sometimes I'd wake up with someone unexpectedly lying beside me and pretend that I knew exactly what was happening so as not to draw attention to my 'drink problem'. This was, for me, the most miserable, tortuous, gut-churning outcome of that thing we call denial. It did not get much worse than sleeping with a man you felt absolutely nothing for, whom you barely knew, and feeling obliged to laugh it off the next morning in order to maintain a pretence that you are, really, actually in control of your life; that you chose to do such a thing.

I am not an alcoholic, I meant to act in this way – I am a free-spirited and liberal woman who enjoys having a good time.

Beneath the lies and pretence was a fractured person living a lie, her insides ripped and hollow, her eyes blank and emotionless. On those occasions I hated myself. When I discuss with people the loss of self-esteem and erosion of confidence as a result of excessive drinking, these are the instances I'm thinking of. I lied to myself, convincingly too, for many years with regards to how terrible many of my drunken actions led me to feel about myself.

I strived for the sexiness of the gently intoxicated woman, but ended up with something far off the mark. Refusing to acknowledge how vile those drunken nights of misguided sexual affection made me feel stemmed from much more than my wish to appear in control of alcohol. I also possessed a deep fear which I never fully appreciated existed as a drinker, that one day I might have to quit boozing altogether. If I accepted how far in the gutter I had fallen, the logical consequence would have been that I should seek help. Getting help equated to stopping drinking. Stopping drinking meant I might learn to be happy, alone – just content, with none of my old props for comfort. And that was a prospect which terrified me.

Carl Jung, the eminent Swiss psychiatrist, wrote a letter to Alcoholics Anonymous founder Bill Wilson in 1961. In this correspondence Jung refers to the craving for alcohol to be "... equivalent, on a low level, of the spiritual thirst of our being for wholeness ..."

This 'thirst for wholeness' is what drives many of us to drink excessively and to utilise sex for the same purpose (as well as becoming addicted to a whole host of other substances and activities such as narcotics and gambling) – a desire to fill an emotional void which yawns and gapes in our hearts like the hungry mouth of a lion. The intangible nature of this void means we aren't always aware of its presence, and even less likely that we recognise how we are engaging in unhealthy behaviours in a desperate attempt to satiate it.

After a great deal of reflection and introspection I am convinced this was the single most influential factor in how I operated as a human being between my teens and mid-thirties. Driven by a powerful urge to fill an unseen void, I drank, smoked, and took drugs, as well as being affected by an eating disorder and a tendency to involve myself in a number of short-term relationships with unsuitable people, with whom I was well matched physically but not in any other respect.

For those who do not feel perpetually compelled to complete themselves via extraneous means, this is no doubt a difficult concept to grasp. I have only become truly aware of possessing an emotional vacuum since I put down the bottle – only then does this affliction rear its powerful head and shout, loudly and incessantly because it is no longer being fed. Carl Jung and Bill Wilson both believed steadfastly that by following religion one could overcome this feeling of emptiness and find comfort and wholeness in God. As referred to in Chapter Two, however, this was not a path I was happy or able to pursue, and therefore I have necessarily had to look elsewhere to discover alternative solutions.

<u>Pregnancy (second time around) and learning to be happy</u>

As I strove to come to terms with attaining inner

completeness minus any god, bad habits, or addictions, I discovered in the August of 2011 (happily I should add) that I was pregnant with Lily. This news came just four months after I had my last alcoholic drink. Body confidence is tested to its limits during the nine months it takes to grow a baby and the subsequent post-partum phase of physical reparation. Pregnancy at the age of twenty-three did not take its toll on my body to anywhere near the extent it did when I repeated the experience at the age of thirty-six. I gained four stone in weight second time around, and the stretch marks which had all but faded since Isobel's arrival (young skin has so much more elasticity!) returned with a vengeance as Lily prepared herself for entry into the world.

I was quite shocked to see my reflection as my weight approached the thirteen stone mark. I looked so different, and felt awful – from extreme morning sickness which gave way to exhaustion, to increasingly chronic insomnia, to piles and cysts and God knows what else; by the time Lily was born I was desperate to get my body back. Walking up a hill has never been as difficult as during the last few weeks of my second pregnancy. The extra weight meant I became breathless on the slightest incline. I would stare jealously at joggers in the park, praying for the day when everything would return to normal and I could begin to enjoy being active once more.

Compounding all of this pregnancy-related unpleasantness was the fact that I ended up having an emergency Caesarean. For any woman lucky enough to have by-passed this procedure, the wound it leaves behind coupled with the lasting drain on energy levels is quite something. For several weeks my abdomen was yellow, blobby, bruised, and lumpen, with a wonky and angry-looking red line sashaying across the lower area criss-crossed with black stitches. For the first week I was bed-ridden, a crying heap of baby blues with enormous milk-leaking breasts and a very unattractive pair of medical stockings which had to be worn to prevent the onset of deep-vein thrombosis. I lost a serious amount of blood during the birth and therefore had little to no energy. My fiancé Sean would inject me with an anti-coagulating medicine every day straight into my blancmange stomach, and I had a colourful concoction of pills by the bedside which I had to swallow each morning with a glass of orange juice (with which to help relieve the obligatory post-birth constipation). After several weeks the Caesarean wound diminished somewhat but it left me with an obvious scar sitting just above the newly reinforced stretch marks.

So there I was, a woman with a history of serious physical self-loathing, someone who had despised her appearance so strongly that she barely ate for the best part of seven years; a person who had not lived one day of her adult life prior to the age of thirty-five (other than during pregnancy and breastfeeding) without either smoking, drinking, taking drugs, or sleeping with Mr Wrong – or frequently on occasion, all four. And a woman who had acted in such a way out of chronically low self-esteem and because she believed she had no real worth as a human being.

Only now, with a tiny newborn baby and a rejection of all the bad habits coupled with a fresh determination to live healthily and happily, I had none of my old crutches to lean on when things became tricky.

Picture this, if you will. I'm standing in a prickly mass of brambles and overgrown weeds, attempting to locate a route out. Leading away from this mini patch of jungle are a number of small paths which all reveal a well-lit and easy-looking means of escape. However, each time I turn to begin walking on any of the pathways, a steel gate slams down before my face and blocks it off as a viable avenue.

In the first year or two of sobriety I increasingly found that my old, tried and tested methods of filling the emotional void were no longer available to me. I might consider buying a bottle of wine after a particularly awful day; bang! Down came the slammer, and a voice bawled at me that I no longer drink. I would turn instead to a consideration of texting an old flame, reigniting the passion for a short-lived burst of excitement and lustful sex; slam! I can't do that any more – I'm responsible now with a new baby and a partner whom I respect and don't want to hurt.

Likewise, drugs and cigarettes had long since fallen by the wayside, and self-imposed starvation was most definitely no longer on my list of unhelpful habits to rely on in moments of crisis (I haven't been significantly troubled by eating issues since Isobel was born in 1999). Left with no quick-fix to turn to I was forced to deal with this hole head on, and, left unfed it became physical, constant, grumbling, and crying out for attention from right inside my heart and stomach (the French expression, *J'ai mal au coeur* literally translates as *My heart hurts* but its true meaning is *I feel nauseated.* I've always felt this to be accurate in the way it points to how our inner core is so comprehensively affected by emotion).

In the throes of early motherhood I was still readjusting to life as a non-drinker, searching for alternative methods (to alcohol) of dealing with stress, anger, and every other emotion, and attempting to discover the sober person's Holy Grail; a means of filling the emotional vacuum. My first major hurdle was learning to accept the noticeable impact pregnancy had made on my body. This is not a disaster when compared to some of the terrible atrocities and tragedies which occur in the world on a daily basis; that I understand. Having a bit of a fat body with a few grim-looking scars and a pair of enormous, veiny boobs never killed anyone. However, with my history of body dysmorphia, one look in the mirror and it was a wonder I didn't collapse in a corner and cry for a month.

But oddly, despite having an increased cause to feel dissatisfied with my appearance I found myself accepting my body image far more readily than I had ever done before. I appreciated the wonder of the female body, and how miraculous the notion is of nurturing a little person inside the womb. I marvelled over the primal instinct that kicks in, in both mother and baby, which establishes a breastfeeding routine. It's true that I hardly stood before the mirror and gasped with delight over my own reflection, but neither did I endure the old negative desires to hurt myself and escape from my own body. I was beginning to like myself again.

In Lily's first months of life I started to understand the natural order of human life, how we must allow time to heal us physically and mentally. I wrapped my head around the way in which we develop emotionally, precisely *because of* events like pregnancy, child birth and the chaos which is thrown up with the arrival of a baby. These are not things we should ever try to hurry along or shy away from. We must live through challenges and difficult emotions if we are to learn and grow.

In my younger years when buckling under the pressures of a warped body image, an eating disorder, and terribly low self-esteem I focused on what was missing in my life as the key to resolving my various problems. If only I was thin, I'd be content. If I had the right boyfriend then I would be fulfilled. If I had more money plus a wider selection of more expensive and fashionable clothes in my wardrobe, I would feel confident and sexy when out socialising. I sought an inner completeness via external means. My outlook on life was fixed, I did not develop in an emotional sense, and I failed to alter any of my behaviour which consistently brought about misery and regret.

Alcohol enveloped me comprehensively from my teens onwards and persistently prevented me from seeing the world as it truly is. But as the sober months passed by in my mid-thirties it was swiftly becoming apparent that as a direct result of becoming alcohol-free I was experiencing a) the reawakening of emotions, good and bad, and b) an innate awareness that this then provides us with an un-blinkered, unfettered perception of the human experience. Suddenly it became clear that for the entirety of my adult existence I had never sought happiness by focusing on me as a person – rather I had always thought I could invite positivity and happiness into my life from purely external factors. In addition I had placed an unnecessary amount of importance on how I looked and had used sex as a distraction, a way of feeling loved and wanted, and as an assertion of my own likeability.

As the world gradually became real again I began to recognise just how far down the wrong path I had ventured in my past efforts to find contentment, not least how I had so often tried to force an outcome of true love out of boozed-up relationships which revolved heavily around sex and nowhere near enough around the stuff that counts.

During the last three and a half years I have stopped despising my appearance, and put the brakes on the forever whirring, negative meanderings of my mind – the terrible, dark thoughts that used to plague me regarding how I looked and how disgusting I once perceived my body to be, have disappeared. As within every other aspect of my new sober life, the thing that has replaced the old adverse self-appraisals is a reality check. OK, I am not Elle Macpherson. I don't like my hair very much and if I'm honest I've never been happy with my nose. But I'm no longer caught in a mental trap where I constantly wish I could vacate my own being and become someone else.

Crucially, I have fostered a positive and proactive approach to life. Whereas the drinking me would have moaned about the way she looked before downing copious amounts of booze to deal with such intensely unfavourable personal assessments, the sober version gets off her butt and attempts to improve things. I eat well and healthily, I don't smoke, I sleep well, I drink lots of water, I have a manicure once a month, I go jogging and to the gym. Making the best of how nature created me now means that I willingly adopt the necessary lifestyle choices for achieving that aim.

Interestingly I have also noticed a massive shift in the role sex plays in my life since quitting drinking. Firstly, I am no longer on the prowl, one eye scanning the near proximity for the next Mr Right, when the current one is standing next to me wondering exactly where he went wrong. Secondly, I do not crave sexual attention or approval of how I look from men I have never previously met. I don't really search too hard for that approval from my fiancé if I'm honest – I prefer him to think I look nice, obviously, and I rather hope he fancies me, but these are no longer obsessive thoughts which rule my every waking moment.

We are busy, and while we love each other, we have a million distractions and chores demanding our attention every day of the week (as do most working parents with young children). I don't need my partner to be within my sight around the clock and he often spends time playing squash, going out on his mountain bike, or visiting the pub with friends, none of which bothers me in the least. This is huge progress for me I should point out, as once upon a time I so despised being left alone in the house that the only possible way I could conceive of enduring the night ahead was to get blind drunk. I would then begin the predictable onslaught of accusatory texting, demanding to know where my partner was, what time he would be home, and who (most importantly) he was with.

Sex, in this far more relaxed and self-confident chapter

of my life, is an act of love. I'm not the raging sex-mad teen or twenty-something I once was, and with a toddler and a hectic work-life balance to maintain, finding the time to be intimate is frequently a challenge. But (a further notable difference to my love life now as opposed to when I drank) when it does happen it is for the right reasons. Sex with the wrong person is not something most people are readily able to fake when they aren't under the influence of mind-altering substances. If one isn't connected emotionally and physically to a person she or he loves then watching paint dry may be a preferred use of time. But, with the right partner and without alcohol screwing things up, screwing can be enjoyed for all the right reasons.

Additionally, because I'm confident that my partner and I share a great deal of mutual respect and trust, the erstwhile motivations for having sex (i.e. making up for a drunken argument or an infidelity, or to reassure myself that he loves me despite niggling doubts) have just faded. I'm no longer manipulative, but honest. I pick up with far greater precision my fiancé's moods; where once a boyfriend's quietness or occasional bout of introversion would have sent me reeling, paranoid and demanding to know exactly what I had done wrong (usually because my memories of the previous night would have been so patchy I wouldn't have known, and thus would be harbouring a suspicion that I'd acted badly in some way), now I just back off and wait for him to talk – if he wants to.

Jumpy, nervous, suspicious, and perennially on the back foot, I was, as a drinker, someone who was unable to put another person before myself. To a large extent this was owing to the fact that as an adult I had always lived under a cloud of fear, awaiting some shocking revelation of 'a terrible thing' I had done during my last drunken episode. A dependency on booze made me into a twisted narcissist, self-absorbed but without any self-love. As a woman who now lives her life in full control of her actions, I've found that thinking of others first comes naturally. I have experienced an enormous sense of relief over the discovery that I am not, in actual fact, a horribly bad and selfish person.

Living free from the shackles of alcohol dependency has sparked a chain reaction of good vibes in relation to how I act within a relationship. My self-esteem has shot up and with it my confidence which has risen to where it should be as a woman in her late thirties. I no longer stutter and stumble over my words, unable to look another person in the eye when I'm speaking and prone to overt blushing. A natural consequence of developing feelings of worth is that I have stopped transferring my hatred of life in general on to my appearance. I view the world, for the most part, as an amazing place, full of opportunity and with the potential to bring us great happiness – living in such a world I no longer find that much wrong with my body or how I look; I'm just real, with all the imperfections of the next woman or man. And with this personal acceptance comes the ability to enjoy a sexual relationship for exactly what it should be; the closest physical manifestation of being in love with another human being. That's it.

Life used to be such a calamitous jumble of problems when I drank alcohol. I was forever struggling with this and that, picking myself up after one disaster before falling headlong into another. Emotions were confusing and relationships a quagmire of guesswork, misunderstandings and lies.

But sober, there is simply me, my family and a lot of real love.

Chapter Seven – Tricks of the Trade

"Advertising is the art of convincing people to spend money they don't have for something they don't need."
– Will Rogers

We are not passive consumers when we wander into the supermarkets but are targeted deliberately by cleverly designed marketing campaigns, and with women forming an increasingly lucrative sector of the alcohol market with the majority of the household purchasing power, we, as females, now constitute particularly attractive customers. Advertising executives are extensively trained, highly paid individuals who have professional psychological insight into how we think, what packaging we will find attractive, which labels we will likely be drawn towards and which film stars will most appeal to us, of vital importance to alcohol manufacturers when considering the various product placement opportunities up for grabs on the silver screen.

There is no doubt that advertising and marketing are incredibly effective and help persuade us in making particular purchases in the booze aisle. If they were not, the alcohol industry would not allocate such astronomical sums to their advertising budgets. In 2001, £181.3 million was spent on alcohol advertising, in comparison with just £75.9 million on soft drinks. The amount spent on promoting alcoholic drinks in 2001 can be broken down in to the following areas: £42.7 million on beer, £18.1

million on spirits and £8.3 million on wine.[14] During the 2000s the annual figure for UK alcohol advertising hovered around the £200 million mark. This, however, is small fry when contrasted with the sums currently thrown at marketing promotions in the UK; £600–800 million per year.[15]

On the Caterer and Hotelkeeper website, an article entitled '*UK wine consumption to hit 151.5 million cases by 2014*' outlines how the UK has become a nation of enthusiastic wine drinkers. The UK is the world's biggest importer of wine, and in 2014 our national wine expenditure is estimated to be in the region of £9 billion. According to the feature, the British public drank 1.765 billion bottles in 2010. This thirst for vino is something which has not escaped the attention of the UK supermarkets. Phil Cave, wine category manager at Morrisons, had this to say on the subject in an interview for *Off Licence News*, the online resource for those working within the alcohol industry:

"Wine for the last two to three years has been acknowledged as a key category where we have an opportunity. That's not changed. The business is putting its money where its mouth is ... We recognised that wine is a major opportunity for Morrisons and invested in it as a major resource. We are seeing positive share development because we are doing a lot of new things and we are now seeing the fruits of that."

As a teenager I had no awareness whatsoever of the way in which I was being manipulated by the alcohol industry. Yes, I was the one who took it upon myself to begin drinking with such vigour but the beverages I

---

[14] Figure from Alcohol Concern Factsheet:
http://www.alcoholconcern.org.uk/assets/files/Publications/Adve
rtising%20factsheet%20April%202004.pdf
[15] Figures from http://www.publications.parliament.uk/pa/cm200
910/cmselect/cmhealth/151/15111.htm#note195

selected, the image I was hoping to portray when sipping them, and certain lifestyle choices in which I felt motivated to engage were all influenced heavily by the way particular drinks were presented to me. My first real favourite tipple was Löwenbräu, the German lager thought to be founded in the late fourteenth century. After Miller Brewing took over American brewing rights in the 1970s, Löwenbräu became associated here and in the US with male bonding, a quality beer of good standing for men who enjoyed the great outdoors. By the time I began frequenting pubs circa 1990 the lager's appeal had shifted slightly towards a younger and cooler audience; it was what all my male friends drank, and I (being the burgeoning ladette) joined in wholeheartedly and sank pints of it every Friday night in a university pub in Sheffield called the West End. As I've said, around that time I also had a taste for 'K', the strong cider which came in a handsome, matt black bottle with the letter 'K' emblazoned in red on the label. The cider was advertised using the slogan: 'Strong. Refreshing. Different' and I remember feeling very grown-up and sophisticated when holding a bottle of it in my hand (although I probably did not look that way after downing a couple, as 'K' was around 8% ABV).

I drank wine as a mid to late teenager only out of necessity – at a party if there was no alternative beverage on offer, or if it was the only stuff my friends and I could lay our hands on when rifling through the contents of a more affluent pal's parents' wine cellar. I would never have bought wine in a pub or nightclub as I associated it with older women, women in their thirties and forties who had careers and husbands, who wore high heels and smart suits. Younger and overly concerned with fashion and image, I opted for the drinks which I felt would provide me with optimum kudos and street cred.

Boddingtons witnessed a surge in popularity during the

1990s and was another drink of choice for me. Tapping into the 'Madchester' music scene, Boddingtons, affectionately referred to as 'Boddies', embarked upon an advertising crusade employing the slogan: 'The Cream of Manchester'. The brewery hired Melanie Sykes in the period of 1996-1999 to front this campaign, a role which sparked her still on-going successful TV career. The Manchester-brewed beer was huge for most of the decade and virtually all the student pubs in Sheffield (the places where I drank most often) sold it. The familiar brewery sign of the yellow-striped beer keg and two bees could be spotted all over the city centre.

I'm certain that I would not have been interested in drinking any type of bitter had it not been portrayed in the way Boddies was. At the time, however, I was unaware of the degree to which I had fallen so easily for clever marketing, believing instead that I was blowing the froth off my creamy beer out of pure choice. The Boddingtons print adverts stood out for their dramatic images of cream-related products like ice cream, whipped cream, and sun cream, all incorporated with a glass of the beer. One of the television commercials featured a couple of Mancunians aboard a gondola, in a parody of the ice cream Cornetto adverts. This, according to the *Manchester Evening News*, "told the world something about the reinvention of the murky old city, that its once-filthy waterway could almost pass for Venice".

Managing director of Whitbread, Miles Templeman, explained that, "We were thinking how to turn a second-rate north-west brand into something more stylish, to make it more appealing again. BBH (Bartle Bogle Hegarty, the advertising agency who created the campaign) thought of focusing on the creamy aspect, of selling a beer like a face cream." These subtle nods to a female market transformed Boddingtons from a local, predominantly male drink, to a fresh and stylish beverage that was drunk readily by men and women alike in their late teens and upwards. The contents remained identical but the sheer power of that campaign demonstrated exactly what it was that we were buying into when we made our pub, restaurant, and supermarket alcohol purchases.

An ex-boyfriend who worked in advertising once told me how at college he was taught to 'Sell the sizzle and not the sausage', or in other words sell the benefits of the product rather than the actual item itself. In his book *Drink*, Iain Gately quotes from *Advertising Age Magazine* in 1984: "More and more it seems that the liquor industry has awakened to the truth. It isn't selling the bottle or the glass or even liquor. It's selling fantasies. Life-style approaches have come into favor as the most effective way for the liquor industry to promote its wares. Psychologically, for consumers to be attracted to these ads, they need to be attracted to the people in them, to identify with the fantasies they create."[16]

The lifestyle approach to alcohol advertising first came into play in the 1980s, and alongside it the industry began to make inroads into cultural and sporting events by way of sponsorship deals across the Western world. Alcohol Concern maintain that there is a growing body of evidence suggesting "… that exposure to alcohol promotion is related to increased levels of consumption, and influences drinking intentions and our perceptions of what we consider to be normal drinking behaviours." Sponsorship arrangements are the epitome of 'selling the sizzle and not the sausage' as they directly link in our minds a particular beverage with, not just an image on a print advert or a brief series of images within a commercial, but an entire event, sometimes lasting days or even weeks, and all the emotions and happy memories that we come to associate

---

[16] Drink, Ian Gately, Gotham Books, 2008, p. 458.

with it.[17]

For instance, Tennent's Lager as the founding partner of the Scottish T in the Park festival has been an active sponsor since the event's inception in 1994. The line-up for the 2014 festival boasts such impressive acts as the Arctic Monkeys, Jake Bugg, Calvin Harris, Elbow, Manic Street Preachers, and Maximo Park, and the event regularly attracts up to 85,000 people. Not only is T in the Park a prime opportunity for alcohol promotion owing to the vast amount of numbers who attend and the media attention which it attracts, but Tennent's has successfully secured its position as a brand which people now associate with music, cool bands, the summer, an outdoor festival atmosphere and all the other connections we make with an event like T in the Park.

The Portman Group (established by the UK's leading alcohol producers for the purpose of promoting responsible drinking and to prevent alcohol misuse) commends Tennent's for its approach to 'safe' drinking in the section of its website on sponsorship; 'Tennent's close partnership with organisers and rights owner DF Concerts ensures that responsible drinking messaging pervades every consumer-facing festival touch point and communication platform from T in the Park advertising, media, promotions, and digital communications to event bar operations and official event platforms to T in The Park.'[18]

---

[17] See http://www.alcoholconcern.org.uk/assets/files/Publication s/Wales%20publications/An%20unhealthy%20mix%20-%20alcohol%20industry%20sponsorship%20of%20sport%20an d%20cultural%20events%20February%202011.pdf

[18] See http://www.portmangroup.org.uk/docs/default-source/sponsorship/t-in-the-park.pdf?sfvrsn=2

People largely attend festivals to listen to live music and drink alcohol. I've been to a few in my time and believe me, if ever you wish to spend time in the company of thousands of people off their face on booze and drugs a festival is the place you should go. Tennent's are all too aware of this fact, hence their enthusiasm to sponsor the festival. However, in order to remain within the government's guidelines regarding the advertising and promotion of alcoholic drinks, the company is mindful to push the 'responsible drinking' message at T in the Park (despite many attendees drinking to excess regardless). 'Responsible drinking' aside (an expression which I find both hypocritical and entirely subjective), the estimated total cost to Scottish society of alcohol misuse in 2006/07 alone stood at approximately £2.25 billion. In comparison, the £60 million sum which the T in the Park festival contributes to the Scottish economy looks like a drop in the ocean.[19]

The widespread sponsorship of sporting and cultural events by alcohol producers has served to ensure that, for many people, attending such occasions is now inextricably linked with getting slightly drunk. Football, cricket, a day at the races; speaking from personal experience, none of these spectator sports when attended by friends of mine would constitute an exciting day out without the crucial ingredient of alcohol. Even people I know who aren't big drinkers in everyday life will adopt the mentality of an ardent boozer when present at a Lady's Day or big football match.

At Doncaster Racecourse situated close to where I live in Sheffield, the hospitality on offer is full of such boozy delights as the Champagne Pavilion Restaurant Package at a cost of £119. This includes admission to the Champagne Pavilion Restaurant, ample food, inclusive drinks, access

---

[19] See http://www.scotland.gov.uk/Publications/2008/05/060915 10/2

to the Champagne Lawn, and a table for the duration of race day. For the lesser price of £73.50 one can purchase the 'Jumps Brunch' package, a deal which incorporates a glass of Bucks Fizz upon arrival. You don't need to search for long on the internet before landing on the pages of companies tapping into the female market who specialise in organising race-day events for hen parties, birthdays, or just for a 'great day out'. All come with the standard 'glass of bubbly' included in the price. As women we are being sold the message that a day at the races necessarily involves donning our glad rags and downing several glasses of fizz.

Far more 'in your face' as far as alcohol promotions go, however, is the blatant sponsorship of the rugby union competition, the Heineken Cup (referred to as the 'H Cup' in France due to alcohol sponsorship restrictions). The Heineken Cup is one of the most prestigious trophies within rugby and is now synonymous with the Dutch lager brand which has been sponsoring the event since 1995. In the American NASCAR (National Association for Stock Car Auto Racing) too, alcohol brands have been prominent as sponsors. The origins of stock car racing can be traced back to the Prohibition period in the United States (drivers largely stemming from the Appalachian region used high-speed cars to transport the illegal moonshine during the dry years of 1920 to 1933), and these days NASCAR is sponsored by Coors Light beer, amongst others. Jack Daniel's whiskey had a sponsorship deal with the Richard Childress Racing 07 car in the NASCAR Sprint Cup Series from 2005 to 2009.

In the sailing world, the America's Cup celebrations have been awash with Moët & Chandon champagne since 1987. In an interview with American publication *The Beverage Journal*, Paige Pedersen, Executive Director of Communications for Moët & Chandon had this to say about the company's role as official sponsor of the sailing competition in 2012: "In sponsoring the America's Cup World Series, we have the opportunity to partner with organizations that share Moët & Chandon's pioneering vision for excellence and spirit of success. Our presence at these sporting events demonstrates our commitment to a race that tests the extraordinary skills of athletes and helps us honor the successes of our past and those we hope to have in the future."

At the 2012 London Olympics Heineken was both sponsor and official lager supplier of the event, a decision which was lambasted by Liberal Democrat MP Greg Mulholland – not, as one might have hoped, for the fact that an alcoholic drink was being linked so overtly to what is primarily a celebration of the physical achievements of human beings. No, Mulholland expressed his disapproval because Heineken is a Dutch firm, saying: "A British brewed beer would be far more appropriate than a Dutch beer for the London Olympic Games."

It should come as no surprise that, in the year preceding the coalition backtracking on its promise to introduce Minimum Unit Pricing, a Commons motion tabled by Greg Mulholland said: "This House expresses its disappointment that Heineken lager, a mass produced non-British beer, has been chosen as the official beer of the London 2012 Olympics, despite beer being the UK's national drink and with the UK being one of the world's leading brewing nations." The current combination of self-regulation (via the Portman Group) and legislation does little to curtail the common perception that excessive alcohol consumption in the UK, whether at home, in the pub, or at a sporting or cultural event is merely a British tradition. Even MPs apparently expressed their disapproval only over the issue of the *nationality* of the sponsoring brewer, rather than the fact that an alcohol brand was being used to represent the London Olympics at all. And when an MP endorses beer as being our national drink, it does pose the question of whether we will ever see tighter regulations with regards to sponsorship and promotions by the alcohol industry.

Prior to quitting drinking, I never regarded the connection we as a society make between alcoholic beverages and sport as odd in any way. So engrained in our behaviour, many people never stop to consider the incongruous nature of this coupling – an addictive, toxic substance on the one hand, responsible for over 2.5 million deaths worldwide according to the World Health Organisation's (WHO) 'Global Status Report on Alcohol and Health'[20], and a variety of sporting activities featuring men and women who are at the peak of physical health and fitness.

When developing their brand image, alcohol producers hone in on the kind of lifestyle and interests which their target audience most aspires to, or those which they can relate to the best. Coors Light (and Jack Daniel's' sponsorship of the Richard Childress Racing 07 car) sponsors NASCAR with the intention of incorporating the sport's image of a daredevil, macho, and all-American approach to life within its own brand identity. Moët & Chandon are keen to hook up with the America's Cup World Series because the sport encompasses luxury, freedom, wealth, bravery, excitement, and elitism – the perfect fit for a champagne brand. Alcohol manufacturers look to support events which bring to life the image they wish to convey for their products, and are fully aware that such associations can be immensely powerful, sticking in our minds for a period far longer than the duration of the event itself.

Lifestyle advertising is not only about partnership with a sporting or cultural event, however. For the last couple

---

[20] See http://www.who.int/substance_abuse/publications/global_alcohol_report/en/index.html

of decades we have also seen an increase in lifestyle advertising in print and television commercials. Blossom Hill wine was, for me, synonymous with friendly female get-togethers (rather than those social occasions which involved serious amounts of alcohol, leading to a state of complete mental obliteration) or everyday drinking; a light and innocuous bottle perfect for that mid-week purchase when I wasn't seeking total inebriation but an easy wind-down after a difficult day. Adverts for this wine consistently targeted the female market and portrayed a group of slim, attractive, middle-class women enjoying girly nights in, always arriving at a friend's house clutching the obligatory bottle of wine, wearing floaty dresses and big smiles. Similarly Nottage Hill and Jacob's Creek were hugely effective in cornering the 'everyday' wine purchase market. An article dated November 2011 in the online marketing magazine, *The Drum*, details a £4.5 million investment package on behalf of Accolade Wines which aimed to boost sales of its Nottage Hill line. Marketing controller at the company, Neil Anderson, states of the campaign; "This significant marketing investment reflects the importance of Hardys Nottage Hill, which has a rich heritage and identity we want to champion, we are confident that the new design, with its substantial marketing support, will help to further drive sales of Hardys Nottage Hill."[21]

Perpetually reinforcing the idea that wine is harmless, trivial, and feminine is the vast array of products that can be found anywhere from supermarket giant Tesco to a pretty little trinket shop in the middle of the countryside. I have witnessed 'A meal without wine is like a day without

---

[21] See http://www.thedrum.com/news/2011/11/18/hardys-nottage-hill-invests-%C2%A345m-promotion-and-new-packaging

sunshine' on a plaque in the gift store of a zoo, and a jokey personalised glass for wine lovers everywhere with the engraving 'Look (enter name here), it's wine o'clock!' available from online gift sellers gettingpersonal.co.uk. In Tesco I have seen on sale a birthday card with the words 'Keep Calm and Carry On Boozing' emblazoned on the front, and each year in the run up to Valentine's Day and Mother's Day, shops everywhere are loaded with bottles of pink champagne and rosé wine presented as perfect gifts for the UK female population at large.

I am not suggesting that the people behind these shopping outlets regularly get their heads together in some kind of conspiratorial secret meeting to ensure that we, the innocent public, continue to buy into the idea that alcohol is a fun treat and something virtually everyone drinks on at least a weekly, if not daily basis. However, the lack of sufficiently tight regulation within the arena of alcohol promotions and advertising results in those with a vested interest having a very long leash indeed when it comes to how they wish to push their alcohol-related products. The overriding impression that we as consumers receive is one of wine being as normal as bread or milk, and that having something of an alcohol dependency (which, let's face it those who use the expression 'wine o'clock' to signal the all-clear for popping a cork are usually leaning towards) is a matter to be giggled over; a 'nudge, nudge, go on let's be naughty' approach to sharing a bottle when there is no especially good reason for doing so. Wine has become the domain of 'normal' mums everywhere in the Western world, nothing more than a pleasant reward for all our hard work juggling careers and kids – and the alcohol industry has much to gain from perpetuating this perception.

Nowhere is this plainer to see than on the website for MommyJuice Wines, the California-based company established by Cheryl Durzy. Durzy is the mother of two children and has a career history in sales and marketing at

Clos LaChance Wines. Her idea for MommyJuice was borne out of the fact that her young children would refer to wine glasses everywhere as containing 'Mommy's Juice', a fact that Durzy admits on the website to finding cute and appealing. The MommyJuice site blatantly suggests that alcohol is an effective coping strategy for parenthood, a message which reinforces the notion that drinking is an acceptable method for dealing with stress and the difficulties of modern-day living. The website explains of Durzy; "Her vision includes balanced, fruit-forward wines that bring just a bit of peace after the chaos of everyday life as a parent." The inference is that wine provides the solution, when in fact it usually exacerbates the issues of depression, stress, and anxiety, all of which are not uncommon in those with young children. In addition, the inclusion of the term 'fruit-forward' implies that these wines are in some way health-giving, fresh, and devoid of the numerous negative consequences of excessive alcohol consumption.

The MommyJuice wines are introduced on the site's home page in the following way; "Being a mom is a constant juggling act. Whether it's playdates and homework, diapers and burp cloths, or finding that perfect balance between work and home, Moms everywhere deserve a break. So tuck your kids into bed, sit down, and have a glass of MommyJuice – because you deserve it!" On a blog contained within the MommyJuice website, Cheryl Durzy explains that she is tired of people accusing her of irresponsibility and that, while she supports those with 'problems with alcohol' there is nothing inherently wrong with her product or the idea of working mothers utilising an addictive, mind-altering substance to cope with the struggles of parenthood. She maintains, "That's it. I have had it with this story about moms and drinking. It comes out every 3–4 months or so, usually when someone is out there promoting an anti-drinking book, web site, program or blog. MommyJuice is almost always a part of it, whether I want it to be or not."

According to the founder of MommyJuice, the stories of women dying prematurely in vaster numbers than ever before as a direct result of consuming excessive alcohol only come to light because someone is promoting an anti-drinking book or website. She purports that accusations wielded towards her company are driven by sexism and that men do not face the same criticisms as women in relation to drinking, asking on her blog, "What does this mean? SEXISM! Yes, this 'moms drink too much' bullshit is totally sexist. I work full time. I take care of my kids. I shop. I cook. I clean. I drown in laundry. I deal with the doctor's appointments, sports, gymnastics, buying birthday presents. There's more, but I am so exhausted from just listing them here I want to fall into bed. Imagine how I feel at the end of a day of DOING? I'm tired and I want to wind down and relax. A glass of wine is a perfect way for me to do so. Men also have wine, beer, scotch. So, my question is, am I supposed to be superwoman and do everything but am not allowed a little relaxation and reward at the end of the day? FML if that's the case!"

I wonder if Durzy has ever visited a liver unit and seen for herself the terrible public health crisis we are facing in the West because of our taste for booze. More than that, if she has ever stopped to consider that by raising our children with the constant sound of wine trickling into a glass in the background, we are instilling in the next generation a normalisation of alcohol as a daily necessity. And if she has considered how sad it is that as capable, grown-up and intelligent women we cannot think of a better more effective way of dealing with stress than numbing our emotions with ethanol, a drug which impedes our ability to think straight, affects our mood, and smothers our intuition and energy levels.

A further example of the way that alcohol is purported to be a thoroughly acceptable and harmless resolution for the struggles we face as working mothers, can be found in the weekly column in Femail (the section of the *Daily Mail* online newspaper which specifically targets women): 'Knackered mothers' wine club by Helen McGinn: A column for every busy woman who's bored of the same old plonk'. This column is ostensibly a wine review piece, but with the added injection of 'humour' and what could be described as a conspiratorial, woman-to-woman undertone which manifests itself in lines such as: "The result is a big, peachy-tasting glassful, with a whiff of lemon peel. Gorgeously crisp too, it'll put a spring in your step even if it's just on your way to the sofa. Food pairing: Chilli-flecked halloumi. Or crisps."

The editorial slant of Femail is one which holds broad appeal – the pages are crammed full of celebrity gossip, beauty and fashion features, as well as information about the latest trends in food and drink. This is mass-market stuff, and the inclusion of McGinn's 'Knackered mothers' wine club' is a direct and powerful acknowledgement of how we, as women, just need to get a glass of wine down us in the evening. It supports wholeheartedly the MommyJuice theorem that life is too crappy to muddle through without a large glass of merlot or a fruity little chardonnay to help iron out the imperfections of our busy worlds.[22]

I have written and spoken openly about my experiences as a regularly drinking parent of a little girl. Having had, since becoming alcohol-free, a second child who has only

---

[22]See http://www.dailymail.co.uk/femail/article-2579899/Knackered-mothers-wine-club-Helen-McGinn-A-column-busy-woman-whos-bored-old-plonk.html#ixzz35eVruw00

ever known her mum as someone who doesn't drink, I've experienced first-hand both lifestyles – sober and not so. I have not brushed away the regrettable times when alcohol took a precedent over the needs of Isobel, and conversely I employ such memories to act as a reminder of one reason why my life (and those of my children) is infinitely better minus booze. When people think of the damage caused by alcohol to families they commonly imagine scenes of domestic violence, or a parent who drinks away the food budget and shouts upon their return from the pub. They might conjure up images of a baby whose basic demands are ignored as Mum and Dad sit in the lounge getting sloshed on vodka or super-strong lager.

What many people do not acknowledge or recognise is the way in which alcohol detrimentally) affects our mood, how the morning after a boozy session we are tired, grumpy, non-communicative, and self-absorbed. The long-term depressive episodes, the manner in which daily drinking prevents us from being as productive as we might otherwise be, and the lethargy which stops us from initiating energetic activities with our children like football in the park or a trip to the swimming pool are all consequences of regular drinking. Over time, each and every one of these affects the way we as parents live our life, and therefore has a direct impact on our families.

However, because we live in an alcohol-centric society which widely supports the idea that booze brings us happiness, success, love, and good times, it is unthinkable to a large percentage of the population that we could manage our lives better if we rebuffed the daily glass or bottle of wine, or skipped the early-evening couple of pints. We are raised on the notion that as adults we *need* to drink alcohol, and brands such as MommyJuice only work towards furthering this belief. The widespread acceptance and celebration of booze in the Western hemisphere is such that to a large extent we have become desensitized to the harms of hazardous drinking. The frequent bursts of coverage in the media pertaining to the UK's binge drinking crisis, the increase in female alcohol consumption as a reaction to the demands of motherhood, and the growing numbers of those admitted to hospital with alcohol-related liver disease – such instances of moral panic originate from a bed of hypocrisy. On the one hand we are berating those who drink to excess, and on the other we are planning our weekend excursions to the pub, or to a wedding which will be saturated with alcohol, or to watch a sporting event where booze adverts will be plastered all around us, or to attend a festival with beer tents and music stages dominated by the logos of alcohol brands.

Any product, whether alcohol, shoes, or perfume, is subject to the same rigorous process of determining who the core target audience is, how best to reach that demographic and which style of packaging and point of sale will ensure the optimum number of sales. And when sales are down, manufacturers will seek to re-examine and reconfigure their original conclusions in order to boost profits. Women, for instance, have failed to warm enthusiastically to the Stella Artois beverage, Cidre, launched on to the UK market in 2011. The cider is described on the Stella Artois website as containing "the full flavour of red apple, enhanced by peachy, apricot notes, complemented by the woody finish." In order to rectify the issue of a dwindling female market, AB Inbev (the global company which owns Stella Artois along with Budweiser and Beck's) has recently introduced a fruity variety of the Cidre drink in female-friendly vessels (apparently we ladies prefer a daintier bottle).

In an article in *Off Licence News* from 2014, Martin Green states that: "AB Inbev has released a new raspberry variant of Stella Artois Cidre in 33cl and 50cl bottles in a bid to attract more female consumers. Nielsen figures show fruit cider value sales tripled between 2011 and 2013, and Ab-Inbev believes the new variant will entice new shoppers into the category. The producer expects women to be more attracted to the 33cl bottles, so it branched off from the traditional 50cl bottle that has dominated the category."

Consumer manipulation is behind every alcoholic product on the market, whether a male-targeted macho brand such as Foster's (the adverts for which are fronted by busty bikini-clad women and lager-loutish, football-crazy men) or a pretty bottle of Babycham adorned with the image of a cartoon-style deer, designed to appeal to the ultra-feminine customer. Babycham, which observed its sixtieth anniversary in 2013, has, according to its website, "… always had sparkle. It has an unrivalled heritage and is always in fashion … It's time to get in the groove with a funky blast from the past because Babycham, the original girlie drink is ready to party." It's easy to see the gender division of the intended audience when comparing this to the Foster's site which constitutes a medley of clips from Alan Partridge and *The Fast Show*, as well as old Foster's TV commercials featuring the aforementioned skimpily clad women, Australian beaches, and dishevelled-looking 'real' blokes who enjoy footy and a pint.

Personal responsibility and social influences

I'm not happy with labelling myself 'an alcoholic'. I do recognise that I have never possessed an off-switch, but I believe it is this together with an untold number of other factors in my life which have combined to ensure I cannot drink alcohol without feeling the need to embark on an almighty bender. My genetic makeup together with the socio-cultural influences by which I was influenced as a child and teenager go a long way towards making me the person I am today. Moreover, we should not downplay the colossal effect that the advertising and marketing of alcoholic drinks has upon the thoughts and behaviours we display as consumers, and how society takes a hegemonic stance on booze as a vital component of virtually all facets of our lives.

Those who feel as though they are in control of their consumption of alcohol and who manage to 'drink responsibly', often express frustration and disapproval with regards to people who regularly drink for intoxication purposes. The former are frequently content to label the latter 'alcoholics', confining them to a part of society reserved for failures, the weak, and the malfunctioning. The stigma attached to people suffering from alcohol-dependency issues is one which follows women particularly closely, and can be difficult to shake no matter what sex one is – a person who was once a regular alcohol misuser may be referred to as a 'recovering alcoholic' twenty or thirty years after he or she sank their final drink. I am opposed to the labelling of human beings in this way as I strongly believe there is a danger of alcohol addiction becoming a person's defining feature; my one-time alcohol misuse does not represent me today and, if it were not for the fact that I run Soberistas, a website for those with alcohol-dependency issues, I would no more give thought to drinking alcohol than I would to snorting cocaine or injecting heroin.

Similarly the word 'alcoholism' is often used when describing the condition of a person addicted to alcohol, but it is a poorly defined concept and one which means different things to different people. The World Health Organisation states of alcoholism that it is "a term of long-standing use and variable meaning", and in 1960, Bill Wilson, denied that alcoholism was a disease, explaining that "technically speaking, it is not a disease entity. For example, there is no such thing as heart disease. Instead there are many separate heart ailments, or combinations of them. It is something like that with alcoholism. Therefore we did not wish to get in wrong with the medical profession by pronouncing alcoholism a disease entity. Therefore we always called it an illness, or a malady – a far safer term for us to use."[23]

In addition to whether or not an agreement has been reached regarding the question of alcoholism being a disease, we live in a world which encompasses a massive range in levels of alcohol usage and dependency. There is the person who drinks a glass or two of sherry at Christmas and barely touches a drop for the rest of the year, and there are the infamous binge drinkers who get smashed each weekend with their friends, pre-loading at home with shots and flavoured vodka concoctions prior to causing mayhem in the city centres. We know of the stressed-out mums, leaning a little too heavily on the evening glass (or three) of white wine, poured after the children have been tucked up in bed. And finally, there is the archetypal drunk, the alcoholic with the red, broken-veined face, a carrier bag full of clinking bottles, shaking hands, and a wreck of a life as a direct result of their addiction.

I would describe my own erstwhile habit as being an amalgamation of the binge drinker and the hazardous drinker, enveloped in a very real state of denial which prevented me from seeking help for many years. On the odd occasion I broached in my own mind the terrible thought that I might be an *alcoholic*, I was aware of a sense of horror, a frightening realisation that I might actually be in a far worse place than I'd previously believed. As I grappled with the term and attempted to locate my own experiences within it, I was filled with the fear that this was what I had become, that despite the years

---

[23] Thomas F. McGovern and William L. White, Alcohol Problems in the United States: Twenty Years of Treatment Perspective, Routledge, 2014, p.7.

of hoping against hope, I had still stumbled and staggered down the one-way road of alcoholism. My life would momentarily appear to be over. And then, because of societal norms and the throwaway comments made by colleagues, friends and family, I would gradually steer away from this newfound belief and come to the alternative conclusion that I was merely a person who liked a drink. I was (as I breathed a deep sigh of relief) still in the camp of the social drinker, the wine lover, the stressed-out mum who had grown up amidst the *Bridget Jones* phenomenon and with *Sex and the City* showing me how grown-up women had a good time. Yes, I may over-indulge on occasion and end up with unexplained bruises on my legs or a half-memory of the night before, but that did not mean I was an alcoholic. I would resume the thinking that my drinking patterns were entirely normal.

When I finally arrived at the decision to quit drinking for good, it didn't take me long to reach the mindset that I did not have an innate disease; that I wasn't vastly different from 'normal' people who are able to 'drink responsibly'. There are personality traits peculiar to me and also to many of those I've spoken to who have found themselves similarly caught in the cycle of dependent drinking, which I believe acted to push me towards seeking a mind-altered state. These include being somewhat sensitive to other people's reactions and worrying a little too much over the way in which someone perceives me, the possession of a creative streak together with a passionate response to the artistic creations of others such as films, music and paintings. I am a perfectionist and very driven, I don't relax easily and I'm very strong-willed. I am at times a loner, finding it uncomfortable and quite stressful to be around people I don't know well. I'm a romantic and a little idealistic, something of a dreamer.

These characteristics combined with a number of

traumatic and upsetting events throughout the course of my life worked towards the development of my emotional dependency upon alcohol. As alcohol is an addictive substance it doesn't take long for our neurological pathways to become hard-wired to craving it once we embark on regular consumption, and certain situations and emotions will then trigger these desires for alcohol more than others if we experience them with greater frequency. For instance, if on every hot summer day we spend time with a particular group of friends sitting in the same beer garden sipping white wine spritzers, soon enough our brains will form the link of: good weather = friends = beer garden = white wine spritzer. Repeated over and over again, this habit will become engrained in our minds.

Certain aspects of my personality, for example being shy around strangers and somewhat sensitive to people's behaviour, propelled me to seek mental escape. If we lived in a world in which heroin was the social drug of choice as opposed to alcohol then no doubt I would have been drawn to that instead. Humans have long sought methods of mental escape, and substances which change the way we perceive our surroundings and alter our mood have held appeal since at least the Neolithic period (circa 10,000 BCE). Scientists working on numerous Neolithic sites across Europe have discovered remnants of cannabis seeds, hallucinogenic mushrooms and opium poppies, suggesting that certain mind-altering substances formed an integral part of the rituals surrounding prehistoric belief systems. However, with the onslaught of sophisticated marketing promotions and clever advertising campaigns for alcoholic beverages thrown into the mix, those of us with a heightened propensity to seek out a means of temporary cerebral departure find ourselves presented with alcohol as the perfect solution – it's cheap, available, and entirely legal.

We are not born 'alcoholics' but I do believe that some

of us have a predilection for excessive alcohol consumption. Childhood influences and the boozy society that we live in are further contributing factors and, in addition, should we be exposed to upsetting or difficult events such as miscarriage, infertility, divorce, bereavement, sexual abuse, or feeling trapped in an unhappy relationship, it is not uncommon to turn to drinking as a means of blotting out the emotional pain. Alcohol dependency then is a continuum, a shifting tendency for heavy drinking that may be borne out of our individual personality traits but which is then affected and moulded by the ever-changing world we inhabit. And should we persist in a pattern of excessive alcohol consumption then we will grow increasingly physically dependent upon it, a state which is perhaps the one we most imagine when considering the term 'alcoholic'.

My choice to not define myself as 'an alcoholic' but a person moulded and shaped by her surroundings who turned to alcohol, an addictive substance, in an effort to self-medicate, is one which assisted me no end in eradicating the shame and burden of stigma which briefly descended in the early months of my new alcohol-free life. Had I assumed the label of 'alcoholic' and proceeded to carry it with me for all eternity, I would not have been able to move forward in the positive way that I have, to focus on the good in me and to concentrate my energies into living as a normal human being who is no longer addicted to anything. It is through education, awareness, self-reflection, and the complete avoidance of alcohol that I've succeeded in rewiring my brain and thinking patterns. Understanding how I have fallen so methodically and predictably for the marketing ploys of the alcohol manufacturers, the ways in which I've been influenced by television programmes, films, and social fashions and fads, and recognising how the government has consistently demonstrated a lack of commitment to strengthening the industry's regulatory boundaries (which in turn would go some way to addressing the dominant societal belief that excessive alcohol consumption is acceptable and normal) – these factors have all played a massive role in reinforcing my decision to live alcohol-free.

The significant impact of the media on our expectations and ideologies most definitely shapes our relationship with alcohol. As we mature into adults our perception of the world becomes criss-crossed with millions of overlapping thoughts and belief systems on everything from the cars we like to our favourite bands to the clothes we choose to wear, and, for most people, the alcoholic drinks they consume. Adverts, the articles in newspapers and magazines, the lyrics in a pop song, an actor's performance in a film; over and over we are targeted with messages which we absorb into our personal take on the world, and which affect the way we interact with everything in it. The media's power to influence is something that we commonly take entirely for granted, failing to recognise just how far removed our lives have become from the way they were just a few decades ago.

In every aspect of life there is a dominant ideology and nowhere is this more obvious than with regards to alcohol. We are told that booze is fun, sexy, and sociable. Drinking is an activity we should indulge in while watching sports, attending a festival, during our time as students at university, on birthdays, when we get engaged and later married, on holiday, at Christmas, at the weekend, in a restaurant, in a pub, at a picnic, at a concert, at the theatre, on a spa day, and at the airport. We are led to believe that alcohol will help us cope with motherhood, fatherhood, relationship breakdowns, to cement friendships, and to make a party go with a bang. Alcohol, we are informed, will oil the cogs of our romantic endeavours, turn men into real men, and will release women from their chaotic lives briefly in order to have a giggly time with the girls. The subtle layers of meaning which are conveyed to us throughout each day are such that we are mostly unaware of the fact that we are being so readily manipulated. Until we realise, one day, that we've been sucked into the middle of a colossal lie – a lie which has brought us to our knees.

Turning away from an alcohol-soaked existence has had many positive effects on me, and has enabled me to become infinitely more aware of the tricks of the alcohol industry. As a non-partaker in this apparently national pastime it has become blindingly clear to me that alcohol is a commodity, as is anything else we can purchase from the supermarket, online, or in the high street. The sole motivation for bringing a new product to market is to tempt the consumer into buying it and it makes no difference if the product in question is an expensive bottle of Waitrose Barolo designed to win over the affections of wine connoisseurs, or if it is a four-pack of Tennent's Super formulated to get the consumer drunk – the bottles and cans are there to maximise profits for the industry despite the fact that alcohol is a harmful substance responsible for damaging millions of people all over the world.

The double standards we as a society apply to drinking result in the alcohol industry largely escaping unscathed in discussions about those who overindulge and venture into the territory of alcohol dependency. When a person is lying in a hospital bed dying of cirrhosis of the liver, or young girls are snapped lying in a city centre gutter with their knickers on display to all and sundry, most will choose to point the finger at the individual rather than the manufacturers of the product which has landed them there. Unlike with cigarettes, in attitudes to which we have witnessed a large-scale shift in recent years, alcohol is still perceived by the majority as being a drug for which the responsibility to consume sensibly lies solely with the drinker.

Labels on bottles of alcoholic drinks bear the words 'Please Drink Responsibly', a message from the UK-wide charity Drinkaware (supported by the drinks industry) which is intended to serve as a reminder to stick within the government guidelines. But the tiny words are so completely and utterly lost in the sea of alcohol promotions and advertising that it is almost comical to expect the consumer to take heed. Seriously, when we live in a world where MommyJuice exists, where an MP describes beer as the UK's national drink and takes exception when a Dutch lager brand is chosen over a British one to sponsor the London 2012 Olympics, when tea-time programming is sandwiched between ad buffers for wine, when a Hollywood film based entirely upon the hilarious consequences of a mammoth drinking session (*The Hangover*, 2009) grosses $467 million worldwide, and when a prestigious rugby trophy is renamed to reflect the lager brand which sponsors it, can we truly be expected to 'drink responsibly'?

Human beings are not robots. Our feelings differ from one person to the next and our reactions to culture and society at large are far from identical. Some of us will feel compelled to experiment with alcohol more than others and go on to use it by way of buoying up our confidence in social situations. Others will seemingly bypass the whole teenage drinking saga, focussing on sport instead and remaining level-headed and steady. Family life can be wonderful for some children, heartbreakingly sad for others leaving mental scars that deepen into adulthood, shaping behaviour into that which is destructive and harmful. Some people's actions will be influenced to a greater degree than others' by the manner in which alcohol is portrayed via advertising and marketing. Taking the view that we are a homogeneous species, all of whom possess the ability to consume alcohol 'responsibly' and who will not, at times, feel a strong desire to escape personal circumstances is naïve and shows a lack of compassion. The stance taken by the alcohol industry is that we as consumers must demonstrate at all times the control required for sensible, moderate drinking – they, after all, provide the message on their products that we should 'drink responsibly'. If we cannot manage this, despite the fact that alcohol is addictive, then we are to blame and should shut up before we ruin the fun of the 'other people' who *are* able to drink in a responsible way.

Raising my awareness over the issue of the alcohol industry's strategies and marketing ploys has enormously helped me to feel happy about my decision to not drink. The key to long-term sobriety is to completely flip one's thinking about alcohol – rather than it being a substance which provides us with all the many benefits extolled by the people who produce the stuff, we must view it for what it truly is; an addictive toxin which kills approximately 2.5 million people worldwide each year,[24] one that causes depression, anxiety, and heightens stress levels, a liquid which when consumed regularly dulls the skin and eyes, is behind blackouts and injuries, which raises testosterone levels in men and women, resulting in violence and angry outbursts, and a highly calorific substance which causes weight gain as well as being the source of feelings of lethargy (which further compounds the issue of weight gain). Perceive alcohol in this way and you will not consider that you are missing out on anything at all.

Becoming savvy about advertising techniques allows us to strip away all the lies and smoke and mirrors surrounding alcohol and therefore enables us to keep focused on reality. When we fail to consciously recognise the manner in which we are being manipulated by the industry, it is all too easy to blithely drift along with

---

[24] See http://www.who.int/substance_abuse/publications/global_alcohol_report/en/index.html

everything we are told, and to keep on merrily downing the stuff that is harming us so seriously. But understanding that every little decision surrounding an alcohol product has been made to ensure the consumer puts their hand into their pocket and parts with their money; how a product is packaged, in which shop it is sold (Waitrose or Lidl?), the price at which it retails, the placement opportunities selected within films, the person fronting the advertising campaign, and the sporting or cultural activity chosen for sponsorship purposes. Understanding of this grants us the power to say no.

Saying no to the alcohol industry's various persuasive strategies contributes towards a sense of empowerment and reinforces the idea that one is *choosing* not to drink, rather than simply *having* to not drink because of suffering from a stigmatised condition. It feels good to stand up to the hegemonic position on alcohol knowing that the blinkers have been removed and you are no longer a pawn in a massive game. I felt exactly the same when I eventually quit my smoking habit – it's a feeling of 'Ha, you're not fooling me any more; I know what you're up to! I'm keeping my money to spend on stuff that won't kill me, asshole!' It's vital to feel in control, to know that you are no longer a powerless sheep trotting along to the supermarket each week and dutifully loading up with bottles of poison that make you fat, destroy your liver, and wreck your relationships.

Reaching this stage of appreciating just how manipulative the alcohol producers are was a massive turning point for me. Not only has it made not drinking easy, but I actually find some perverse pleasure in exposing this pervasive untruth; alcohol does not give us anything other than the temporary respite from a craving. Yes, we know there are people out there who are capable of 'drinking responsibly' and that's all well and good, but I'm talking to YOU – the person without the off-switch, the one who has been made to feel guilt-ridden and shit because you cannot stop after one drink, the person who has struggled to work out whether you are an 'alcoholic', the person who desperately wants to escape the booze trap. Regaining a sense of control in a world filled with companies seeking to alter your behaviour to suit their financial targets will help you stay strong in the wine aisle.

Learning to say no to alcohol is immense – it will mark the beginning of a whole different way of life, where you can feel good about being kind to yourself. And it will really piss off the fat cats of the booze world.

Chapter Eight – The World is a Better Place Sober

"I have just three things to teach: simplicity, patience, compassion. These three are your greatest treasures."
– Lao Tzu

Stopping drinking for me has amounted to an experience which runs much deeper than merely opting for a soft drink when I'm out with friends, or no longer spending extended periods perusing the various bottles on display in the supermarket wine aisle. Becoming alcohol-free has changed me from the inside out, dramatically altering my perspective on both myself and the world around me.

I am fully aware of why booze remains so attractive to a large proportion of the population. There are numerous reasons why alcohol eventually became problematic for me, but nevertheless, I did have some good times when drinking; I enjoyed the instant feeling of relaxation it provided me with, the ease of alcohol-fuelled social interactions, and the manner in which it curtailed my perspective on the future.

This last point is something which I never recognised as taking place at the time but with hindsight I can see occurred all too readily. My focus was usually restricted to the next drinking opportunity, and consequently I rarely considered my existence beyond a few days ahead. This resulted in me never overthinking the idea of my own mortality (other than on those occasions when I'd wake up in the middle of the night plagued with fears over developing breast cancer or cirrhosis of the liver) or the meaning of life, or how I, as an individual, could make the most of my time on Earth. In limiting my thoughts to the immediate future I managed to avoid any deep consideration of life or death. To a large degree, booze allowed me to bury my head in the sand and not become excessively troubled by the certainty of mortality.

But although I wouldn't dismiss the sum total of my drinking history as a *complete* waste of time, I am without doubt that my life is immeasurably better minus its presence. In the last three and a half years I have learned so much about human happiness, about my own emotions, my plus points and shortcomings, and what it takes for me to be fulfilled and happy. It has not been a straightforward journey and many a time I've flirted momentarily with the notion that perhaps I *could* have a drink; that maybe the old issues surrounding moderation and dependence wouldn't resurface. It was, for a while, a two-steps-forward-one-step-back road to contentment, but I have now arrived at a place where I know I'll remain for ever.

The most monumental difference in me since becoming alcohol-free can be located in my new-found ability to live in the moment. Mindfulness constitutes the cornerstone of Buddhism and for followers of the religion it is the key to a happy life. I seem to have stumbled upon this way of living purely by accident as a natural consequence of putting an end to my alcohol consumption, but it is *the* core reason behind my ongoing commitment to a sober lifestyle and shouldn't be underestimated in terms of its importance for achieving a state of emotional calm.

So what exactly is mindfulness, other than something which allows us to remain in the present? Put simply, it enables us to steer our way out of the tangle of thoughts that fills our heads most of the time. Mindfulness stems from ancient Eastern philosophies central to both Taoism in China and Zen in Japan (in addition to Buddhism). It is frequently linked to the practice of yoga, and has grown in popularity in the West over the last few years. More and more people are coming to realise that mindfulness is inordinately effective as a method of controlling their feelings, even when they are experiencing hardships. It is about letting go of worry and fear, abandoning our anxieties about what might be around the corner and no longer affording time to extensively mull over past behaviour. One might regard mindfulness as emotional awareness, a heightened self-knowledge which, when mastered, brings about the opportunity to halt negative thinking patterns in their tracks in order to fully appreciate being in the present moment.

Believed to be the author of the short book *Daodejing* (or *Tao-te ching*, commonly translated as the "Classic of the Way and Virtue"), Lao Tzu, or Laozi, was a Chinese figure generally considered to have lived during the sixth century BCE. [25] He was intrinsic to both the philosophical tradition and the organised religion strands of Taoism. Laozi's book is the most translated work of literature after the Bible, and places emphasis on the Dao as the source of all existence. The Dao is interpreted as 'The Way', of which wu-wei (action through non-action) is the core ethical principle. Wu-wei stresses the importance of existing in an uncontrived manner; of 'going with the flow' and avoiding any attempts to defy the natural order. It promotes the idea of living in harmony with the universe, in the manner of the tree which grows without conscious thought or a river that flows without premeditation to do so. In fact, in original Taoist texts, wu-wei is frequently associated with water because of the latter's yielding yet powerful properties.

Buddhism teaches that by increasing our emotional intelligence and encouraging the mind to be more selective in the thoughts on which it focuses, we can bypass many of the excessive negative feelings that often determine the

---

[25] Although some suggest he is dated to the fifth or even fourth century BCE.

course of our life. This mental fine tuning is achieved through meditation and mindfulness. The essence of these Eastern practices is to reach a stage of fluidity in the mind – to zone in on the here and now and to avoid becoming caught up in any fears of the future or regrets over the past. By concentrating on the present and ensuring we devote our attention fully to whichever activity we are currently engaged in, we can ditch the vast majority of our less helpful thinking.

It can be incredibly empowering to arrive at the realisation that a thought is nothing more than an opinion, a way of interpreting an event rather than a statement of fact. For instance, if a person receives a poor assessment from her boss of the work she has done, she may perceive this as meaning she is no good, unintelligent, and less capable than her colleagues. These thoughts might then become pervasive, obstructing other more positive ones from entering her mind and reducing her motivation, level of effort, and overall self-confidence. However, the original conclusions drawn from the words of her boss are not fact but a mere opinion that she has chosen to believe. As an alternative, this member of staff might opt to interpret their boss's dressing-down as a sign of weakness on the boss's part; the boss failed to provide adequate instruction, or, for whatever reason, has a personal vendetta against the staff member. Either way, these opposing justifications for the behaviour of the boss are nothing more than thoughts, opinions, or competing versions of the same event.

Practising mindfulness means that we train our mind to pay attention to *actual experience* rather than our mind's interpretation of that experience. Pema Chödrön, Buddhist author and teacher, wrote, "If someone comes along and shoots an arrow into your heart, it's fruitless to stand there and yell at the person. It would be much better to turn your attention to the fact that there's an arrow in your heart ..."[26] This is a helpful reminder of the importance of living in the moment, but it also highlights a characteristic with which many of us are imbued.

Wasted effort expended on emotions which serve no purpose is commonplace in British culture. As a society, we frequently fail to demonstrate gratitude for that which we have, focusing instead on the things we deem to be wrong with or missing from our lives. With stress constituting a major cause of physical and mental disease, we can be quick to experience anger and upset over the most trivial of things, and this is manifested in numerous situations, from road rage to shouting loudly at our children for acting up in public. As a people we often seem to be very busy, highly strung, and not especially skilled at relaxation – unless it involves alcohol.

Anyone who has ever hit the bottle too hard on a regular basis will recognise the inherent features of a heavy drinker – the regrets, self-loathing, shame, and embarrassment caused by our behaviour when under the influence. I estimate that for each hour I spent drinking alcohol, I must have spent an equal length of time the next day agonising over my drunken actions, the connected health risks I was facing, or simply how rotten I felt owing to my hangover. Every day, following a binge, I would hide away indoors agonising under multiple waves of self-disgust and fear. In addition, I allotted much headspace to needless worries and anxieties over some imagined future dilemma, usually money-related. I had no awareness whatsoever of the idea that I could control what was springing up in my mind, and so I allowed myself to be bruised and battered by a steady onslaught of terrible, uncompassionate thoughts.

The further I distance myself from my old boozy existence, the more I appreciate the wisdom of Lao Tzu

---

[26] Start Where You Are: A Guide to Compassionate Living, Pema Chödrön, Element, 2003.

and other ancient Eastern philosophers. Lao Tzu outlined simplicity, patience, and compassion as the three greatest treasures of mankind; speaking from personal experience, I possessed these characteristics in limited amounts as a drinker. Since becoming alcohol-free I haven't made any special effort to embrace a simpler existence or to be a more patient or compassionate person, but how I approach day-to-day life has completely altered in a very organic way. And at the forefront of this transformation are simplified expectations and the vast reduction of the constant elasticity of my thought processes.

In the old days my thoughts would bounce about in my head like lively frogs – my mind was a constant churning mass of fears, worries, and negativity. Everything was based on an 'if' or a 'when'; *'when I've finished these chores I can go to the pub'*, or *'if I can make it through to the end of the week without alcohol I'll reward myself with a bottle of wine on Friday'*. I almost never enjoyed the actual moment I was living in, as I spent virtually my whole life wishing away the present in order to reach the point where I could legitimately pour an alcoholic drink. And then when I finally arrived at the stage where I was lifting glass to mouth on the verge of enjoying the beverage I'd been salivating over for the last few hours, all I could think of was whether there would be enough to last the night. For a split second in between popping the cork and relishing the sound of the liquid as it hit the base of the glass, I was present in my life. And then, bang! The thoughts would revert back into overdrive mode and my mind would speed ahead to the future – *'there's only a couple of glasses left'* and *'is it bad to buy a second bottle on a week night?'*

When our minds are preoccupied with what has happened before or what might occur in the future, we are not experiencing life – instead we are consumed by stories, fears, and fantasies which may or may not be close to the truth, but which, in any case, almost certainly occlude the mind's ability to appreciate the here and now. Right now is, in fact, the only thing we have; it is the sole absolute truth in life. Learning how to bat off the bombardment of ideas regarding the past and the future, the chain reaction of negative thinking patterns, is vital if we are to enjoy that which is real and unencumbered by ego, fear, or regret.

Adopting mindfulness has caused my old tendencies of overcomplicating life to diminish substantially, and I now seek to simplify things wherever possible. The apparently banal or tedious has become joyful and/or satisfying. For example, carrying my fitful toddler around her bedroom late at night in an effort to rock her back to sleep is no longer perceived as a chore or an exercise in frustration. As a drinker I would have viewed such a situation as one which prevented me from being elsewhere, namely the lounge with a glass of wine to hand, or standing on the doorstep with a cigarette and a beer. My erstwhile addiction to alcohol resulted in me wishing away any instances in life which acted as a barrier to an unhampered access to booze, and I often struggled to hide my irritations on such occasions.

In the same scenario but minus the alcohol, I'm left to concentrate on my little girl's wellness, and spending an hour singing softly in an effort to help her drift back off to sleep is considered no hardship at all. I'm not trying to escape, mentally or physically, and as a consequence I am calm and compassionate; this more positive reaction then transfers to my daughter, helping her to reach a state of contentment more easily. I am better able to focus on the present moment because I'm not continuously yearning for an addictive substance – nowadays there *is* nothing more important than the moment.

My past relationships (and the first few months of the one with Sean when I still regularly drank alcohol) were all affected by my insecurities and inability to trust. As a result of an incident which happened to me at the age of twenty, I was beset by a morbid fear of being alone in the house. Lying semi-naked in the spare bed at a friend's house one summer's night back in 1995, I awoke to discover my ex-boyfriend standing over me wielding a hammer. He proceeded to drag me by my hair from the bed, out of the door, and along the corridor where he urinated over me and kicked me. He then pulled me down a short flight of stairs and hauled me outside, locking the door before jumping into his van and driving away with a screech of tyres. I was left lying on the ground, stunned and frightened for my life.

Unbeknown to me, the house I'd been staying in had been empty, the owner having left after I'd fallen asleep to go clubbing for the night. My ex, knowing that I lay sleeping inside, had shinned up a drainpipe and climbed in through the window which he'd smashed with his hammer. It was five o'clock in the morning, and I made my way to the nearest public phone box to call the police, still semi-naked and my skin sticky with urine.

This nightmarish scene was to consume me for months if not years to come. I was terrified of being alone, my drinking escalated, and ultimately I moved to London for several months in order to seek a safe haven from the man who was still boldly roaming the streets of Sheffield, untarnished by his horrific actions of that night. For well over a decade after the incident, I was filled with fear whenever I found myself in a house as the only adult – something which caused problems in all my subsequent relationships, and which led me to self-medicate with wine as a routine measure if such an occasion ever arose. Boyfriends were regularly subjected to drunken pleas to cut short their night out and return to keep me safe from imagined intruders. Upon them informing me in the first instance that they were planning a night out I would try every trick in the book to ensure they stayed at home to protect me.

I understood why I acted in this way, as did the majority of my past partners, but I found it impossible to shake the terror that would fill me at the very thought of being in the house alone. This was a classic case of allowing the mind to completely take over one's life, to the point of rendering me to the verge of a mental breakdown. The horror stories I dreamt up would spiral wildly out of control; the slightest noise was indicative of a burglar, shadows told a thousand tales of lurking prowlers who crouched in the dark until they saw the perfect opportunity to attack.

Believing these fantasies meant that I felt compelled to seek external relief in an effort to dampen the resultant fears – relief brought about by wine. The numbing property of alcohol put an end temporarily to the rising panic which criss-crossed its way through every last corner of my mind, although it also stifled every other emotion in the process. Eventually I would drop off on the settee late at night, waking in the morning with a crippling hangover but my anxieties mollified with the knowledge that daylight had arrived and I hadn't been attacked during the night.

Many people in the West, myself included prior to 2011, spend their entire lives swayed by the whispering stories which fill their mind. In being held captive to often illogical, rampant thought processes which influence us to act in particular ways, we are never living in the moment and are overcomplicating our lives unnecessarily by listening to fantasies that will never come to fruition.

There is an inextricable link between the practice of mindfulness and overcoming addiction, which is that by heightening our emotional intelligence we can successfully separate the 'addict' voice from our rational minds. Whether you call this voice the Wine Witch, Vodka Vampire, Wolfie or anything else, you'll be aware of exactly what I'm talking about if you've ever lived through a craving for alcohol.

The incessant internal chatter of the addict voice can be heard intermittently, breaking through the wall of 'normal' thinking in its efforts to convince us that we should have a drink. So ignorant was I of this phenomenon as a drinker that I genuinely mistook the Wine Witch as a part of my own cognitive workings for over twenty years. I thought that it was *me* who was pondering the issues of whether I had a problem with booze, was an alcoholic, could ever learn to moderate or whether or not there was any problem with excessive drinking in the first place – after all, don't we all partake in the odd boozy session now and then? The voice was so real and seemed such an inherent part of me that I never considered for a second the possibility of distancing myself from it, or that I could choose to ignore its persistent prattling.

In the early days of living AF, my addict voice was loud and difficult to discount – it almost hurt physically to power through its persuasiveness with my own rational voice, the one that exists free from any external stimuli or addictions. But over time this little war of the minds grew less arduous, and certainly after a year or so, opting to overlook the addict's views on anything became second nature. The Wine Witch may have popped up out of nowhere (usually on a sunny day when I'd witnessed droves of happy-looking people sipping alcoholic drinks in a flowery beer garden) but I could quickly and easily push her away with the self-assured spiel of my own true voice – the one which recognised the lies and rose-tinted-glasses view of the alcohol addict who still remained (albeit in an ever-decreasing form).

In dealing with my alcohol-related thoughts in this way, the practice of mindfulness and certain Taoist principles have gradually and naturally encroached on all other areas of my life. Coping with eight solid weeks of extreme colic episodes in my newborn baby (complete with projectile vomiting several times a day, and four hours of relentless screaming every evening between 7 p.m. and 11 p.m. – the baby, not me) provided me with evidence enough of how capable I had become at eliminating endless streams of negative and angry thoughts. As soon as I began to feel stressed and wound-up by thinking of all the chores I'd yet to finish, I would bring my focus back to the present and forget about everything else. It was pointless expending mental energy on the jobs waiting for me while Lily was in so much pain – remaining calm and measured would only serve to help her settle more readily, consequently enabling me to take care of other matters sooner (like going to bed!)

Practising mindfulness has brought about, again without any real concerted effort, a leaning towards a more simplified existence. Mindfulness demands an appreciation of the apparently more mundane aspects of the world, which in turn has reduced my desire to fill my life with endless 'stuff': new clothes, shoes, bags, make-up, cushions, crockery sets, and gadgets are no longer perceived as items capable of filling an emotional hole. They are practical purchases, bought if and when required but never because I am looking to them as a means of making me happy. I'm more likely to buy something after thinking about it first for a few weeks, as opposed to making impetuous purchases that are soon to be relegated to the back of the wardrobe or kitchen cupboard.

I used to visit the supermarket almost every day owing to the fact that I never found a spare hour in which to plan the week's meals and create the associated shopping list. Incidentally, I think visiting with such frequency also provided me with a sneaky back-up plan with regards to last-minute wine-buying whenever I feared supplies at home were running low. Shopping with such regularity eroded at least five hours of the week, and the meals we ate as a result of not forward planning were usually based on convenience or processed foods. Now, with more time on my hands (because I don't drink) and no need to make up excuses to visit the supermarket (to disguise sneaky wine purchasing), I put aside an hour at the weekend to plan the week's meals. I write a list, one of us (Sean or I) goes shopping, and we save ourselves a lot of time and money – and eat far healthier meals. Mindfulness has prompted me and my family to eat in a more intelligent way.

Somehow and without me even noticing, I have conquered my deep-seated fear of being home alone in the evenings. When I am on my own these days, I actually enjoy it – the quiet, having sole control over the TV, not having to consider anyone else's feelings for a rare few hours. The doors are locked and our dog will bark if someone tries to break in, and that's as far as I ever go with regards to thinking about intruders. Several years ago I would not have believed that I'd be able to sit on my own in a house, stone cold sober, and not be crippled by fear, downing multiple bottles of wine. But it has just happened. Neither would I have imagined that a Friday or Saturday night could pass by without a single word from the Wine Witch but this is now my usual weekend experience.

The central tenet of Buddhism is that we cannot obtain happiness from outside of ourselves and that life will undoubtedly throw unpleasantness at us, but it *is* within our control to maintain an inner peace if only we can let go of the mind's delusions. Buddha is generally understood to mean 'Awakened One', as in a person who has awakened from ignorance and who therefore sees the world and everything in it as it really is. A Buddha knows not to believe thoughts and delusions which arise on an almost constant basis, and recognises that neither positive nor negative emotions are true reflections of the external world but constructions of the mind.

I should point out that I am neither a Buddhist nor a Daoist but that there are strands of these ancient belief systems that really work for me, when incorporated into my atheist experience of life. Meditation has been an enormous help in improving my ability to ignore the addict's voice in my head, and in addition it calms me when I feel stressed. Mindfulness is most definitely a practice which I cannot see me abandoning – it's become engrained in the way I live, every minute of every day, and has enabled me to notice the true wonder of the world around me in a way I never did previously. In addition, I am fond of the Daoist principle of wu-wei, to strive to work with life as opposed to against it, and to be more accepting of certain truths.

My first real awareness of Taoism came about in my late teens when it was introduced to me by a friend as we sat in a chairlift high above the French Alps. The lift had temporarily broken, leaving everyone riding on it suspended in mid-air for approximately half an hour until the engineers managed to get things moving again. My immediate reaction was one of panic – at more than 2000 metres above sea level and a fear of heights this predicament did not sit easily with me. And then my wise friend began telling me about Taoism, how we can aim to accept a situation and look for the positives in it, rather than struggling to fight against that which is immovable. I looked around me and absorbed the incredible views of icy peaks, snow-covered chalets and the bright blue sky, and understood. We were so lucky to be there, and I still remember that beautiful scene now as if it was last week.

Unfortunately, heavy drinking had a habit of muddying the waters of my mind, and so this Taoist precept was one which I failed to incorporate into life with any kind of regularity – at least until I quit the booze.

I am fully aware nowadays of when my mind strains to return to the old habit of winding itself up faster and faster, the thoughts and ideas spewing out in a complete free for all. This, I cannot believe, I once accepted as merely the way I was – an intrinsic element of my personality over which I had no control. I even justified my excessive drinking as a method of instilling some calm to the whole crazy proceedings in my head; that somehow it was 'allowed' for me to down a bottle or more a night as I suffered from an overactive mind. Who knew there was such an easy, healthy and totally free way of managing this modern-day Western malaise of monkey-mindedness?

In the first few weeks and months after I stopped drinking, I often internally debated the notion of religion, conscious as I was of the emotional vacuum that had unfurled within me. After almost three and a half years without alcohol I have now come to a place of understanding with regards to this sense of there being something missing. I have a tendency to fear the future – nothing catastrophic that may be years down the line but usually some imagined situation later on in the same day. It's a low-level panic which can lead me to believing problems will arise should I pursue a particular course of action. Faced with the proposition of, '*Shall we get a babysitter and go out for a meal tonight?*', my thoughts can automatically become concerned with potential difficulties; my parents might be too tired or busy to want to babysit, Lily could be ill or impossible to settle, I may be exhausted and need an early night.

Once upon a time, pre-mindfulness, I would have very easily allowed myself to be influenced by this stream of negativity to the point that I'd have refused to leave the house. This established itself as fairly customary back in my first sober year. However, I am now acutely aware of this mental process as it begins to take place and refuse to accommodate such negative ideas, employing mindfulness as a method which prevents things from running amok in my head.

As a drinker I suffered exactly the same spiralling, negative thinking patterns but as a remedial measure I would pour myself a glass (or three) of wine. This was effective (in the short term) in putting an end to my immediate fears or anxieties and I'd feel more relaxed and able to face whatever it was that my mind was obviously struggling with. This old tradition of constantly using wine as a means of shushing my worries was, I believe, the very thing that led me to feeling so adrift in those first few weeks off the booze. Because I was still in the early stages of becoming accustomed to an alcohol-free life, I had yet to sharpen my emotional awareness and therefore didn't fully know myself.

Unable to focus on the present moment, I conceded to drift along with the fearful thoughts in my head, and consequently felt frozen with fear over quite the most innocent of situations. It was like being caught in quicksand; although I desperately wanted to act in a free, unencumbered manner, I was held fast by a series of imagined problems and heightened levels of anxiety. I craved, more than anything, a strong entity to hold me and prevent me from falling into the chasm of self-doubt. There was a sensation of freefalling, of terror over an unknown future – as though my imagination persistently leapt one step ahead deliberately, simply to force me into a permanent state of uncertainty.

This feeling of being too loose, too free in the world, caused me to lean towards thoughts of religion. If I couldn't rely on my old protector, wine, then I would need an alternative source of comfort, and unable to see that the problem lay *within* me, I was attempting to locate this extraneously. It is clear to me now that at the time I had a very profound desire to be looked after, of being unable to operate as an independent adult.

Looking to alcohol to curtail escalating negative thought patterns may appear to work at the very time of drinking. We feel a degree of emotional numbness almost as soon as we take that first sip, and a blessed sense of relief derived from the cessation of the whirling mental gymnastics. But for anyone who wishes to be free of the endless cycle of dependency on this addictive substance, who wants to enjoy living in the moment instead of constantly looking ahead or behind, mindfulness is the secret to a calmer, more fulfilling existence. Ultimately, alcohol only serves to compound our anxieties.

Referring back to Chade-Meng Tan, Google's 'Jolly Good Fellow', he once said, "Success and failure are emotional and physiological experiences. We need to deal with them in a way that is present and calm." And this is the key to a happy life, as I see it now. There is no point in allowing our minds to become trapped in a permanent state of thought-surfing, where one idea links to another, and another, and then to a whole series of wild fantasies, none of which is ever likely to happen in real life and therefore serve no purpose at all. Wasted thought lifts us out of the present, to which we can never revisit. And for me, overthinking always dragged me down into a state of relentless anxiety from which I found it an almost insurmountable task to escape.

Remember the earlier analogy of the person who's had an arrow shot through the heart? It is of far greater worth to focus on the arrow than on the person who fired it.

Compassion and humility

The ego is responsible for mediating between the conscious and the unconscious mind; it is the backbone of who we think we are and our individual interpretation of reality. When I was at my lowest ebb, my own ego grew to mammoth proportions. At a time when my self-esteem (balanced, positive self-love and respect) was reduced to virtually nothing, my ego exploded into a giant, manipulative monster that would stop at little to attain even the most miniscule signs of approval and validation from others. So terrified was I of being considered a nobody, unworthy and unloved, my ego took it upon itself to ensure that people stood up and noticed me, and at the height of my destructive relationship with booze this facet of my personality was at its very worst. An inflated ego is not borne out of feelings of self-worth, but a fear of not being good enough.

When we are weighed down with the negative mental and physical effects of excessive alcohol consumption, the injection of false confidence obtained through drinking can lead to hubris. As our self-esteem is depleted through the constant battering of regrettable boozy behaviour, the ego often attempts to counteract the situation by growing in size. It thrives on anxieties and fear over not being liked, feeding off feelings of shame and unworthiness. And when our sense of self becomes unbalanced in this way, emotions such as anger and jealousy develop, creating further problems. In my own experience, the emphasis was always predominantly on others and how they perceived me – my expectations and (often wrong) assumptions of their words or actions frequently led me to feel depressed and unloved.

Several years ago, prior to becoming alcohol-free, I was not sufficiently mentally stable to distinguish between these different features of my mind – the ego, self-esteem, and self-image were concepts to which I did not devote any thinking time. I simply was who I was. But I see things very clearly now with the clarity gained through being sober and am aware of how, with a healthy ego and self-esteem, a person usually demonstrates compassion more readily than they do without. Sobriety has granted me humility, a characteristic I was consistently lacking as a drinker. The Indian-American author and physician, Deepak Chopra, maintains that, "We must go beyond the constant clamour of ego, beyond the tools of logic and reason, to the still, calm place within us: the realm of the soul." Being a non-drinker for three and a half years has brought me to a place where I finally grasp what Chopra means.

Many people will emphasise hitting their rock bottom as *the* major motivator that was required to stop them drinking for good. This is certainly how things panned out for me, although I would hate to wish my own story on anyone else, and there are plenty of people who successfully and permanently quit drinking without having been though a terrible booze-related incident. However, as far as my own story goes, I'm convinced that the violent aftershocks which followed the last time I drank alcohol laid the essential groundwork for my happy commitment to AF life.

I'd actually been giving a lot of thought to quitting drinking during the weeks leading up to that night, but for whatever reason on that particular Wednesday I fancied a bottle of wine. I already had one chilling in the fridge and so, once I'd finished with dinner, I settled down with a magazine and a large glass of icy cold pinot grigio. My daughter was staying the night with her dad and therefore I felt entirely free to indulge in a session of guilt-free boozing – alone and away from prying eyes was, by then, my favourite type of drinking. After about an hour I had drained the contents of that first bottle, and so wandered up to my local Tesco in order to buy another. Clutching a bottle in my hand as I stood in the queue waiting to pay, my eyes were drawn to a display in the chiller cabinet where a 'Buy one get one free' offer jumped out at me. I hastily swapped my one bottle for two of the promotional variety, paid and left (holding the bag as still as possible to prevent embarrassing clanking – how I do not miss any of that!)

The hours which ensued are ones that are mostly

missing from memory. I vaguely recall taking a litre of vintage cider from the fridge after I'd drunk both the additional bottles of wine, but everything is blank after that point. And so it was with utter confusion and self-disgust that I awoke many hours later in a hospital bed in Sheffield's Northern General Hospital, my clothes cold and sticky with congealed vomit and a bright light staring me in the face. I do not have to try especially hard to remember how I felt physically – the churning stomach, unbelievably pounding headache and that revolting taste initiated by excessive alcohol and vomit, all spring vividly to mind with little effort.

I was informed by my friend (who probably saved my life by discovering me on the pavement and calling an ambulance) of everything that had taken place, and was discharged by a duty nurse who had obviously seen this type of thing once too often. After reaching my apartment I showered, put my pyjamas, on and crawled into bed where I cried for what seemed like an eternity.

Many things ran through my mind as I lay curled up in bed with Betty the dog. Probably first and foremost was the startling realisation that I would never be able to drink again. The penny had finally dropped and I knew that I would never be able to manage my alcohol intake should I, at any stage in the future, allow myself to swallow just one sip. Christ, I thought. A life sober – that's a biggie. More fundamental, though, was the way in which my ego had splintered into a million fragments, leaving me with the sense of having nothing; no soul, no heart, no control, no history, no future, no purpose, no idea of who I was. I literally felt as though I was nothing, a hollow husk, and that the grand total of virtually all the experiences I'd lived through to date were of absolutely no value. I was the end result of twenty years spent running away from myself. I felt very strongly that I wanted to give up and die.

Over the course of the next few days, things eased

slightly, and I began to look ahead once more in an effort to work out how to live, now that Mr Pinot Grigio had been consigned to the recycling bin for good. I regard my last night of drinking as being monumental, a real turning point which allowed me to wipe the slate clean and start again – fresh and a little bit wiser. Over time, I began to see how all my priorities had been severely misplaced, how self-centred I was. I vowed to overturn my personality, a process which had already begun with me waking up in the hospital bed and finding a sense of humility for the first time in my whole adult life.

Sigmund Freud once said, "A man should not strive to eliminate his complexes but to get into accord with them: they are legitimately what directs his conduct in the world." This statement is of great magnitude to the person who is seeking to successfully walk away from an alcohol dependency. Humans are complex beings and our behaviour is determined by the intricately interwoven elements of the mind. Drinking alcohol brought about such a degree of negativity with regards to how I once perceived myself that, with my self-esteem scraping on the floor, my ego went into overdrive in its attempts to locate signs of reassurance, evidence that I was loved and well-liked. But with an increase in my emotional intelligence, I've found the strength to look inwards for validation. Learning to depend on myself for a sense of calm and perspective has eradicated those old fears of being unanchored and in need of protection. The world is not so frightening when you are tuned in to reality and confident in your ability to manage your thoughts.

Since becoming alcohol-free, I've become far more aware of my ego, noticing when it is beginning to step out of line. Nowadays when I feel insecure, for example, I am able to remove myself from the situation; take a step back, meditate on whatever the issue is that has caused my upset, and recalibrate my perception on the world. I reign in the thoughts that have begun to ravel again, I question my actions – am I in the right? Could it be that I have jumped the gun or been unfair? I reconnect with that feeling of humility, that I am no bigger or smaller than any other person on the planet. I am an equal.

Lao Tzu said that, "Mastering others is strength. Mastering yourself is true power." With the clarity brought about by a non-drinking lifestyle, it becomes less challenging to know and assess one's own mind. Separating the various strands of it and grasping how we can continue to develop positively has become a way of life for me. The more time I spend sorting myself out mentally, the better I am able to take on the obstacles that life is guaranteed to throw my way intermittently. A return to simple values, a healthy and active lifestyle, and a commitment to live in the moment without becoming preoccupied with trivialities and fantasies, all go a long way to removing one's self from the madness and internal chaos of a life defined by heavy drinking.

"You build on failure. You use it as a stepping stone. Close the door on the past. You don't try to forget the mistakes, but you don't dwell on it. You don't let it have any of your energy, or any of your time, or any of your space." – Johnny Cash

Chapter Nine – After the Storm

"I look to the future because that's where I'm going to spend the rest of my life."
– George F. Burns

I have moved a vast distance from the person who decided in April 2011 that it might not be a bad idea to quit drinking. When I look at old photos of myself I can't quite believe that the woman featured in a variety of scenes that almost always featured alcohol, is me. Other than the fact that I am now older we don't look too dissimilar in appearance, but I am fully aware of how very different we are on the inside.

What's changed? Put quite simply, I now think of matters other than alcohol. Visiting a friend's house is an occasion no longer overshadowed by obsessive thoughts of whether wine will be on the agenda, coupled with a discreet perusal of the kitchen sideboard – are there any bottles? How many? Will they be opened, and when? When the sun shines, my thoughts turn, not to getting drunk in a beer garden but to a walk in the countryside, a game of football in the park with my toddler, or enjoying an ice cream with my family as we sit beside the local boating lake. Friday evenings no longer signal the onslaught of a mammoth drinking session during which I will poison my body with countless alcoholic drinks, cigarettes, and a hefty dose of shameful behaviour. The weekends now mean relaxing, winding down, and looking after my body and mind.

For me, switching to an alcohol-free life was all about

discovering how to ditch the booze without becoming a miserable non-drinker. I had no interest whatsoever in a 'one day at a time' approach to life, where I could conceive only of making it through the next few hours without wine but tomorrow might be a whole different ball game. (It should be noted, however, that approaching a life minus alcohol in the early days is all about short-term, manageable chunks of time, and I certainly worked through the early weeks on a 'just for today' basis). I didn't want to change much either, transforming into a boring do-gooder who frowned at the excesses of others and tutted when she witnessed a group of heavy drinkers getting sloshed. Neither did I want the rest of my life to be defined by the fact that once upon a time I drank too much. I just wanted to be a normal person, who doesn't drink alcohol.

Since becoming a non-drinker I've journeyed through an extensive range of emotions and perspectives regarding this new chapter of my life. Right at the very start I was scared stiff and stifled with depression over losing the substance which I considered my best friend. I was filled with terror over missing those quiet evenings in; just me and a bottle, when I would get lost in the blackness of my drunken mind and indulge in the soothing effects of addressing my addiction. I imagined an endless, dreary existence ahead without the crazy, reckless nights out, the debauchery and the rock 'n' roll life, the gratuitous pleasure-seeking. I perceived my entire personality as having been bundled up and tipped onto a rubbish heap – the old Lucy was gone, and God only knew who was coming to fill her shoes.

Later on in that first year off the sauce I found myself growing increasingly angry and bitter; why the hell could everyone else get pissed whenever they fancied it while I was suddenly confined to the part of society reserved for boring old farts? I was a dry drunk, wishing I could get hammered but employing sheer willpower instead to steer myself away from the wine aisle and the pub. Those few months were my worst fears realised – it was what I had dreaded the most, and to make matters worse, it was also the period during which my mind chose to process a variety of painful past events.

My divorce, friends who had fallen by the wayside because I was a selfish wino who couldn't be bothered with nurturing relationships, difficult emotions surrounding my erstwhile eating disorder, and truckloads of guilt regarding Isobel and how, on numerous occasions, I had not been terribly responsible as a mother; it all rose up like a tsunami, knocking me to the floor in a wave of remorse and prolonged emotional wretchedness. Simultaneously, I despised every person on the planet who was able to drink alcohol 'normally'.

Thankfully this was merely a phase, and by the spring of 2012 I was definitely beginning to emerge out of my cocoon of self-pity. I have to credit 'Juicemaster' Jason Vale with changing the course of my life, for after reading *How to Kick the Drink ... Easily!* around this time (as recommended to me by a friend who had also ditched the booze after years of social binge-drinking), I experienced a total overhaul in the way I regarded alcohol. In addition, this book brought about many questions in my mind surrounding the people, myself included, who are labelled 'alcoholics' by society at large.

What is it about this substance, I wondered, which means that consumed in small to moderate amounts it's viewed as entirely acceptable – actually, more than that; drinking up to the point of becoming overtly drunk is encouraged, glamorised, revered, and considered sophisticated. Even inebriation is something we tolerate, so long as it's 'funny drunk', 'weekend drunk', 'wedding drunk', 'Christmas drunk', 'World Cup Final drunk', 'birthday drunk', and 'birth of baby drunk'. But as soon as a person oversteps the invisible parameter and steps into the dark, terrible world of 'alcoholism', everything changes.

Instantly it becomes a pity game, a prison of labels and fallen reputation. A non-drinking 'alcoholic' is deemed to be for ever 'in recovery', a person who didn't know when to put the brakes on like 'the rest of us', someone who faces a future of secret meetings, mineral water and God, in an effort to ensure she never again picks up a drink.

Why is alcohol viewed in this manner, when heroin, tobacco, cocaine, and ecstasy are not? I took ecstasy, coke, LSD, marijuana, speed, and magic mushrooms on a fairly regular basis during my mid to late teens. I was emotionally dependent on these recreational drugs since I was, deep down, consumed by unhappiness and low self-esteem, thus I ingested them to escape my reality – plus pretty much everyone in my social circle also took them, so it appeared rather normal. I enjoyed some good times when taking these drugs, and likewise they caused me a certain degree of mental and physical discomfort on occasion; bad comedowns and bad trips are as integral to drug-taking as the hangover is to drinking.

Gradually, as I grew older and the rave scene could no longer hold claim to the zeitgeist, I stopped taking drugs. Many years later, I do not consider myself as being 'in recovery' from these substances, merely that back in my teens I took a few drugs. Neither do I regard myself as being 'in recovery' from alcohol today. It is an issue of semantics, but this was *my* problem, and the language I utilise to write or talk about it has been an essential element of how I've managed to become a happy individual who is not weighed down by a one-time dependency upon booze.

Alcohol is thought and spoken of differently from illegal drugs because it is so widely consumed by everyone, from kids on street corners to prime ministers and presidents. It is *the* accepted drug of choice. The very people seeking to address the harms wielded by this drug drink it too, and the politicians who enact laws intended to control its usage are also known to consume it. As a society we do not think of this as strange, although we may well regard it as utterly bizarre if we hypothetically slot an illegal drug into the position of alcohol, as it features in society today. Occasionally I find myself doing this; an apparently innocuous advert for booze appears on the television and I wonder how we would feel if this was an advert for heroin, or cocaine. The layer upon layer of normalisation that has ring-fenced booze from this kind of scrutiny, however, ensures its stance as a totally socially acceptable addictive drug.

Reading Jason Vale's book made me question whether I was comfortable with bearing the label of 'alcoholic' for ever, if indeed at all. I realised fairly instantly that pigeonholing myself in this fashion would only add to the already quite severe levels of shame and embarrassment I was feeling. I do believe that I qualify as a human being who can, and *should*, be defined by her character and actions of the present time, and *not* by an addictive substance on which she became reliant during a period of her life. I also believe passionately that, rather than sobriety being perceived as an almost apologetic lifestyle, it should be aspirational; a very positive path to follow.

Ever since I dropped the 'alcoholic' label I felt good about not drinking. Being completely sober has evolved in my mind as a major part of who I am, of which I am inordinately proud. I love not drinking, and I love everything that goes alongside this lifestyle choice. I no longer drool when I observe others boozing, and I hate it when people act awkwardly around me purely because they feel uncomfortable about the fact that I don't drink. A few people have expressed real sympathy towards me since I stopped drinking, a phenomenon that I put down to how we, as a society, regard 'alcoholism'. I've felt the arm of a person I hardly know around my shoulders, as they have asked me, 'And how are you – now?', as if they were speaking to a teenager rather than a grown woman. I've received apologies expressed by those who are enjoying an alcoholic drink, worried over my reaction as if I might feel compelled to lurch forwards to grab their glass and throw its contents down my neck.

The hypocrisy and misunderstandings can be as massive on the sober side of an alcohol dependency as in the drunken thick of it. People generally do not wish to examine their own drinking behaviours, and many feel somewhat defensive towards how much, and how often, they consume alcohol. I know several people whom I would classify as hazardous drinkers and who have extended the hand of sympathy towards me upon discovering that I once had a 'drink problem'. Yet when I socialised with them as a drinker and they witnessed first-hand my drunken shenanigans, there were no concerns voiced whatsoever.

However one chooses to define one's self is, of course, an entirely personal matter. There is no right way, only the way that is right for each individual. But for me, 'Soberista' is a much better fit than 'alcoholic'.

I like the word 'Soberista'. I refer to myself as a Soberista, and I'm proud of my life and the choices I've made in it. In focusing on what you wish to become as opposed to that which you are seeking to leave behind, you are denying alcohol any more of your attention. To me, being a Soberista means that I choose to live without alcohol because I have learnt that my life is happier and healthier without it; it symbolises the shift I've made from a person who persistently ran away from herself, to someone who faces life head on, no excuses. It's a massive deal, to recognise that you cannot and probably will never, be able to moderate – becoming a Soberista has enabled me to fully accept that fact and to feel content at being free of alcohol.

Not drinking alcohol has affected a noticeable change in me with regards to how deeply I consider the world. Virtually all my spare time once revolved around alcohol and this meant that every activity I engaged in was either a precursor to drinking, or the actual piss-up. For instance, when I ran the Sheffield half marathon in 2002, I crossed the finish line, grabbed my medal, and then me and my group of supporters immediately hot-footed it to the pub where I sank several pints of lager. A day trip to London would amount to a reluctant trawl around a few sights (not particularly paying attention to anything) prior to finding a bar somewhere in Soho, where me and whoever I was with would proceed to get hammered. A train journey equated to an uninterrupted drinking session meaning I neglected to notice the scenery outside, or appreciate the available quiet time perfect for dissecting a newspaper.

The many benefits that I have found in being AF are, to me, what it is to be a Soberista. This way of life is about being present and appreciating your life fully; it's about having the clarity and intuition to recognise where things could be improved, and possessing the energy required for initiating any necessary changes; it means being totally in tune with yourself and your emotions, and living in closer proximity to a natural, non-toxic state. To adopt the term 'Soberista' is to celebrate all of these benefits, and in doing so I have been able to detach myself and my experiences from the negative connotations often associated with the word 'alcoholic'. For me, life is about the present, not where I was several years ago.

Ironically, one of my goals when I quit drinking was to embrace a novel chapter of my life in which I got to live as a person untroubled by booze – to be one of those people I once regarded as slightly strange, who never crave any mind-altering substances to make it through the day. As the founder of Soberistas.com, however, my whole existence now revolves around alcohol. I write about it, talk about it, and read about it, every day. I have become far more aware than I was previously of the terrible damage that this drug causes; how wretched it makes those who are dependent on it feel, and the vast burden of shame and ill health people suffer at its hands. I have delved into the murky world of the alcohol industry and been shocked and appalled by the amount of power they possess, and the freedom they are granted to market their products.

But I'll be forever grateful that certain factors in my life led to the creation of Soberistas and that its existence has brought together thousands of people who've connected with one another, arriving at the realisation that it isn't only them lacking an off switch. Soberistas, on a very personal level, has shown me that there are masses of people, from all across the world, who have felt the same despair I once did; that there are great numbers who are seeking a happy and healthy life without alcohol and who feel compelled to fight against the associated stigma and prejudice. The thousands on Soberistas are evidence that there are changes afoot in our society, that we aren't all content with being drunken bums who blunder through life with a bottle never far from reach; they prove that lives *can* be turned around and that a person who commits to sobriety can and should feel pride and contentment as a result of their lifestyle choice.

My biggest fear in stopping drinking alcohol was that my soul would die. I simply could not conceive of living without booze as it seemed that every last iota of my being was linked in some way to drinking. In the same way that smoking once provided me with a physical reinforcement to the image I wanted to portray (rebel, rock 'n' roll), alcohol gradually became the embodiment of all that I was – or, at least, all that I imagined I was. In the first phase of sobriety I felt as though my entire personality had been sucked out of me.

I can see now, though, that alcohol had previously formed such a major part of my whole life experience that, for a while as a sober person, absolutely *everything* appeared odd. Just over three years later and with the dust having finally settled in my new, booze-free landscape, I know that my soul didn't die – my addiction to alcohol died instead.

The facets of my character which I believed represented the person I was and all that I stood for have turned out to be nothing more than manifestations of a fairly intense dependency upon alcohol. Those traits were borne out of a twisted and poisoned mind, one which was moulded by the toxic effects of ethanol and all the resultant emotional consequences thereof. Low self-esteem and confidence, shame, guilt, and regret; these were the factors that helped shape my personality and they all stemmed from drinking far too much, for far too long.

Put very simply, removing alcohol from my life has cleansed my soul. What is left behind is a Soberista.

The Nine Precepts of the Happy Soberista

1.   There is nothing to fear from starting afresh – life is a series of learning curves. The successful Soberista learns from their mistakes and isn't afraid of trying again.

2.   Wino to Soberista is not usually an overnight transition. Be gentle on yourself and recognise that you're growing in strength every day – admitting you have a problem is the first, and most important step.

3.   We can choose the language we employ to talk about our experiences with alcohol – everyone is different and that is perfectly OK.

4.   Alcohol does not have the power to define you; it may alter your behaviour as it negatively affects your mind and body, but beneath that façade is the genuine, and best, version of you.

5.   Living alcohol-free allows us to engage honestly with others, appreciate fully our surroundings, and become properly acquainted with our inner self.

6.   There is only right now – mastering the mind eliminates fear and anxieties over that of which we have no control; the past and the future.

7.   Compassion puts the brakes on an expanding ego.

8.   Happiness begins with a guilt-free mind.

9.   You are number one – the wellness of your loved ones stems from your own, so never neglect yourself.

Bibliography:

Books

A Fiction of the Past, The Sixties in American History. Dominic Cavallo, Palgrave, New York, 1999

A Talent for Humanity, Ros Black, Anthony Rowe Publishing, 2010

Alcohol Nation, Aric Sigman, Piatkus, 2011

Beauty for Ashes, Lady Henry Somerset, Gill, 1913.

Drink, The Intimate Relationship Between Women and Alcohol. Ann Dowsett Johnston, Fourth Estate, London, 2013

Frances E. Willard, Let Something Good Be Said: Speeches and Writings of Frances E. Willard, Chicago: University of Illinois Press, 2007

Start Where You Are: A Guide to Compassionate Living, Pema Chödrön, Element, 2003.

Websites

http://www.adventist.org/information/official-statements/statements/article/go/0/chemical-use-abuse-and-dependency/36/

British Medical Journal
http://jech.bmj.com/search?fulltext=shipton+alcohol&submit=yes&x=0&y=0

Joseph Rowntree Foundation Report –
http://www.jrf.org.uk/sites/files/jrf/UK-alcohol-trends-FULL.pdf

http://www.theguardian.com/lifeandstyle/wordofmouth/2014/feb/24/which-band-beer-top-of-the-hops

Cancer Research UK
http://scienceblog.cancerresearchuk.org/2011/02/04/why-are-breast-cancer-rates-increasing/.

Alcohol Concern UK
http://www.alcoholconcern.org.uk/campaign/statistics-on-alcohol

http://www.cdc.gov/nchhstp/newsroom/docs/STDs-Women-042011.pdf

http://www.guardian.co.uk/lifeandstyle/2012/dec/27/women-weight-minister-jo-swinson

http://www.pbs.org/wgbh/amex/missamerica/sfeature/sf_list.html

Alcohol Concern Factsheet:
http://www.alcoholconcern.org.uk/assets/files/Publications/Advertising%20factsheet%20April%202004.pdf

http://www.publications.parliament.uk/pa/cm200910/cmselect/cmhealth/151/15111.htm#note195

http://www.who.int/substance_abuse/publications/global_alcohol_report/en/index.html
http://www.thedrum.com/news/2011/11/18/hardys-nottage-hill-invests-%C2%A345m-promotion-and-new-packaging

Quote from Andrew Langford, CEO of the British Liver Trust

"Many of us, whether female or male, will be able to identify with a lot of Lucy's experiences; her honesty and openness provide a stark insight into how easily people become dependent on alcohol and get hooked on what our society (and that means each of us) has allowed to become our most harmful commodity.

The World Health Organisation recognises that "Alcohol consumption is the world's third largest risk factor for disease and disability; in middle-income countries, it is the greatest risk. Alcohol is a causal factor in 60 types of diseases and injuries and a component cause in 200 others." Lucy's words portray a very personal picture of what this means but we all have a responsibility to take stock of how we are allowing alcohol to create so much personal and societal damage.

Good Luck to all Soberistas – your commitment to a healthier lifestyle is an enormous credit to all of you.'

Other titles you may enjoy

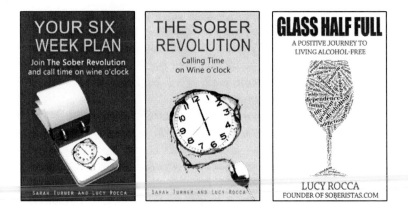

For more information about **Lucy Rocca**

and other **Accent Press** titles

please visit

www.accentpress.co.uk

For news on Accent Press authors and upcoming titles
please visit

http://accenthub.com/

Lightning Source UK Ltd.
Milton Keynes UK
UKOW04f2146060315

247427UK00001B/5/P